Laugh Your

Abs Off!

The hilarious way to lose
weight…forever!

By Tim Wilkins

Stand-up comedian, trainer, and
award-winning healthy TV Chef

Laugh Your

Abs Off!

**The hilarious way to lose
weight…forever!**

By Tim Wilkins

ISBN: 0615783260

ISBN-13: 978-0615783260

DEDICATION

To my wife Michelle, who continues to say in word and deed, "I can do it!"

And to my amazing family who are like a protein shake, blended, and making me stronger every day.

Contents

Introduction

I'm sure we can all say without hesitation that dieting sucks. In fact, the only thing worse than dieting is dieting over and over, only to lose weight and gain it all back...plus *more*.

Some people, let's call them freaks, actually have no problem living every day on what most would call a "diet." They eat grilled this and steamed that, and tasty sauces are either put "on the side" or left off completely. These freaks are a waiter's nightmare and make everyone at the table feel guilty when they order.

They're even worse to be around at the pool. Heaven forbid you lay out next to one of *those* people with their flat stomachs and their thighs that don't touch. You almost want to wait until they fall asleep, and then write "bitch" in suntan lotion across their six-pack abs!

For the rest of us, however, it takes a combination of willpower, planning, kicking, and screaming to unpack the junk from our trunks.

After all, pizza is delicious, nachos are much better loaded, and supersizing makes good financial sense. Right?

I could go at this like most diet books with stats, facts, and figures about obesity and heart disease, blah, blah, blah, but you've heard it all before.

You know being overweight is unhealthy, and who wouldn't like to look fit and feel good? "Look fit and feel good," there's the first joke in the book. Being overly skinny isn't the answer, either, so there has to be a middle-ground between looking like Jennifer Aniston and being on Jenny Craig.

Most of us would just like to put on our favorite pair of jeans without sprawling across the bed and using pliers to zip them. Of course, if you are one of those people who are only a few tools and a little elbow grease away from actually wearing your favorite pants, you probably aren't in any big hurry to make lifestyle changes. I guess that's why they call those jeans "Lucky."

This is actually how most of us gauge our weight, with degrees of fashion that let us know where we are without ever stepping foot on a scale. Our wardrobes contain several types of clothes that function like warning signs, similar to the terror alert colors the government created.

They start with a few pairs of "Wow, do I look good in these!" pants. Next comes the majority of our clothes, which fall into the "I guess I could live like this if I had to" category. The last batch consists of a few outfits made out of stretchy material which finally forces us to admit to ourselves, "It's time to do something about my weight."

It's not just the size of our clothes that tells us these things, however. The makers of bigger clothes still haven't figured out how to make all that print or color look as good as the "little" ones. The result is that when you are wearing your "big" clothes, you look like you're wearing either a bedspread from a cheap motel or an over-sized Skittle.

The partnership between food companies and the media certainly doesn't make things easy for us to stay in shape, either. All of their marketing dollars and slick ad campaigns lead us to foods that are bad for us. "Eat this candy bar and get more energy." "Drink this beer for a better life." You never see a commercial that says, "Eat broccoli, get laid" or "People who like oatmeal wear gold watches and drive fine German automobiles."

The average person has tried at least four times to lose weight, so don't feel badly if that includes you. And if you've tried more times than that, then you are actually above average. Great job!

Rather than beat yourself up over failing, however, think about the fact that you are still trying.

We all dream about changing, but it can come down to trying again and again, until we find what works for us to make that change stick. I think a good example for us all would be that Hugh

Heffner keeps getting married. On the surface, this appears to be about finding love and happiness, but the reality is that his under-aged wife du jour thinks she will change his philandering ways, when all Heff really wants is someone hot to change his silk *Depends*!

When it comes to what you might have tried so far, have you joined a club in which you meet once a week with other people who are miserable about their weight? Good times, right? Bonding over flavorless diet chocolates and complaining about how much weight you *haven't* lost has definitely got to be near the top of your "to-don't" list.

One of my favorites is the dieting plan that includes "windows" with little pictures of the foods you can have for the day. When you eat a food, you close the window. It's nice in theory, but you know what they say: When a window closes, a refrigerator door opens.

Or maybe you joined a club in which they took the guesswork out of eating by providing what they (but not *you*) considered to be "meals"?

The only problem with their plan was the food tasted like it came from a hospital cafeteria, and when you peeled back the foil on their packages, you prayed that what you saw was just the appetizer!

Maybe you became *really* desperate to get in shape for a big event like a class reunion or a wedding, and you tried starving yourself or living on warm lemon water and carrot sticks. Of course, you lost enough water weight to get into your tux or hideous bridesmaid's dress, but you felt more tired and cranky than your menopausal high school gym teacher with the too-short hair and a man's name.

You might even have fallen for the latest magic pill meant to burn fat while you sleep. Unfortunately, it made you more jittery than a toddler on a Halloween candy buzz, and you got *no* sleep during which to burn fat. After a frazzled week of living like a crackhead with insomnia, you stopped taking *Snooze-it-off* and left it in the medicine cabinet until you saw on TV that the FDA was pulling it from the store shelves for killing a half-dozen people.

None of this works. I know it, you know it, and the diet industry knows it. Yet they make billions every year preying on our desire to get in shape by selling us quick-fix trash and books touting magic cures.

These books only lead us, still overweight and hungry, back to the book store, where they now sell coffee and muffins. We can't catch a break!

Too many people think they can just go on a temporary diet, because that's what they are hoping will do the trick. These people (not *you*, of course!) think if they can just avoid certain foods for a while and lose a little weight, they can go back to their old ways of eating. Wrong! You can't go back. Grab my hand, Carol Ann…stay away from the light!

So what are we supposed to do? Know this, first: Eating right needs to be a way of life that happens consistently over the majority of your life. There are no quick-fixes! The only way you are going to lose a lot of *unwanted weight* overnight and keep it off is if you go through a divorce. And even that can take 60 to 90 days, depending on how much you have to lose.

The next thing to accept is that diet success has to start with the right attitude. I suggest that we choose laughter, because the process of changing over to a healthier eating style is probably going to be about as much fun as that little "exam" we all have when we turn 50. Thumbs up, if you've already had it!

You know from experience that as soon as you start eating "healthy," you're going to be hungry. At your first thought of starting a new eating plan, junk food stars in an ongoing dirty movie in your head. Asleep and awake, you fantasize about fried food, chips, and whatever else you normally crave.

You want to call people during dinner and ask, "What are you eating?" in a breathy, stalker voice. And, oh, what you are dying to do to that donut hole…! That's because the first things that come to mind for most people who think about eating healthy are starvation, deprivation, bland food, and general misery.

Many of those points, such as the food being a little plain at first, might be true. Diet food is not necessarily bland, like what you eat when you visit Nana in the Old Folks Home and she insists you stay for dinner, but it's mostly pretty boring. However, the real reason that diet food might seem like it's missing a little zip is because it won't be filled with that fat/sugar/salt-bomb that was in your previously scheduled go-straight-to-your-ass processed and fast food.

Throughout this book, I will own up a few times to the fact that grease, salt, and sugar (which give us that nifty carbohydrate high we get from huge portions of pasta, rice, and potatoes) are delicious, but they are making us FAT! They are also deadly. So, it's time to break the addiction and move on to a new way of thinking about food, dropping a few choice pounds in the process.

This book is a culmination of 20+ years of combining comedy with diet and health knowledge. My ultimate dream is that you:

- Have a really good time reading it

- Learn useful things from it

- Actually *practice* some of what you learn, in order to lead a healthier life

I'm going to do my best to stick to the theme of ripping up all of the BS you've been fed about diets and exercise, and follow that up with some useful information. The book is full of tips, tricks, and, although it's subjective, comedy. If you laugh hard and hold your stomach in really tight, I promise you'll have six-pack abs*. The most important lesson to be gained here is that losing weight and living healthy is a *lot* easier than we're making it.

(*Training equipment, nutritional supplements, personal trainers and chefs, steroids, liposuction, tanning beds, and anything else needed to accomplish this goal is not included. Promise not valid in countries where fast food is sold.

And, believe me, the only guaranteed way to have a six-pack under your shirt is if you shoplift beer.)

About the Author

What the Heck is a Fitness Comedian?

I don't know if doing comedy came about as a result of getting picked on, or I got picked on because of my smart mouth. At this point, it really doesn't matter; it's kind of a "which came first, the chicken or the egg white?" thing. I know for sure, though, that in addition wanting to be a standup comedian when I grew up, my other dream was just to *grow*.

Besides being beaten on, it was being the last one picked for the kickball team and the one the girls talked to about their boy problems that gave me the inspiration to seriously hit the gym.

I started lifting weights around the age of 16, and was quickly hooked. The first muscle group to develop was my back, the lats, as the gym rats call them. They stuck out from my body like wings, and my sister said that I looked like a maxi-pad.

Thinking back, she might have said mini-pad. But in *my* mind, I was a big, buff feminine hygiene product, a regular Kotex the Barbarian!

A couple of years later, I entered my first bodybuilding show, easily winning the title of Mr. Teen Gold Coast. All right, so there was no one else in my weight class, but I waxed my parts for that show and, for me, that was harder than the training and dieting. (Think Chewbacca in a banana hammock; how's that for an appetite suppressant?)

I did well in my next few shows, even with competition, and seemed to be transitioning nicely from Arnold Drummond to Arnold Schwarznegger. I thought, "How cool is a sport where people clap for you in your underwear?" But before my professional muscle career could seriously launch, bad genetics and the even larger dream of being a comedian continued to gnaw at me.

So I put my clothes on and headed to the comedy clubs in the hope of getting people to laugh *with*

me while I was wearing clothes, rather than *at* me.
I worked the amateur circuit across Southern
California by night, while paying the bills by
working at my buddy Derek's gym by day. His
gym happened to be down the street from one of
the biggest bodybuilding magazine publishers in
the world, so there were photo shoots with pro
bodybuilders being done there regularly, which
was really motivating.

The first time that my two dreams intersected, I
got to be in a magazine spread with one of my
idols, the Incredible Hulk. It was called "Going
Rep for Rep with Lou Ferrigno is no joke!" Being
included in that article was one of the most
exciting things that had happened to me in my life,
regardless of the fact that even at around 200 lbs.,
I looked like Little Sprout next to the Green Giant.

Not long after that, the comedy bookings started
to outweigh the glamour of being a trainer, and I
was off to pursue the bright lights of the stage.
Don't get me wrong; it was a hard decision. I
almost had to flip a coin to make a choice between
performing in Las Vegas for an audience of

thousands and getting up before dawn to count to 10 for people who weren't any happier to be there than I was! I managed to break away from training, though, and didn't get another chance to help people change their bodies (or help myself change mine), until almost 10 years later.

When I first started getting work as a comedian, I had no idea what the reality of being a touring "road" comic would be. It quickly took a toll on my physique. We've all watched hugely obese people on TV being removed through the windows in their homes and taken to the hospital on whale stretchers. And, as we watched, we condescendingly wondered why at some point they didn't notice how much weight they were gaining, and felt certain that could never happen to us.

The truth is that it could. In fact, I transitioned fairly easily from obsessed with fitness to drifting into fatness.

For me, the day of reckoning came when I was getting my car serviced. I was driving a lot on the

comedy circuit, and had taken my car in for yet
another oil change. While I was hanging out in the
waiting room, I stood next to a life-size image of
the Michelin man and saw an uncanny
resemblance between him and me in our reflection
in a pair of hubcaps. "It's got to be the shape of
the rims," I told myself. "They distort images, like
a circus mirror." But, no. Sadly, what I saw was
the *real* me, pasty, white, and full of spare tires.

It made sense, though, because my diet had gotten
pretty bad. The combination of the budget I was
on as a struggling comic and my heavy travel
schedule had me eating in places with drive-thru
windows and signs like, Truckers Welcome. And
we all know that when money is tight, there is no
better way to stretch a dollar than gorging yourself
at cheap buffets.

However, that quickly leads to wearing stretch
pants and clothes with brand names that start with
"Big" and "Lane."

If I'd been trying to break into TV as a "before"
shot for a diet commercial, my plan would have

been right on track. (Years later, I was beaten to *that* dream by my friend Larry the Cable Guy, who took the diet company gig for a while until saying, "Screw it!" and signing on with a heartburn medicine instead. All I can say is, "Git' er done, Larry!")

Realizing that where I ate was based on how much I had to spend and that wasn't going to change, I did some research on how I could get the best bang for my nutritional buck at the grease outposts at which I was limited to eating. So I went to work mapping out places where I could get high-protein, low-fat, balanced meals for breakfast, lunch, and dinner.

I also found that, dedicated as I was to my goal, it was still next to impossible to fill all of my nutritional needs while I was on the "McRoad." So I turned to supplements as the solution, and started stocking up on protein bars and shakes, more or less turning my car into a rolling GNC. I even traveled with a blender and a George Foreman Grill for a while. When my career got to the point that most of my traveling was done by plane, the bars and shakes stayed in my luggage, but the small appliances were left behind.

I did this because of the new TSA standards and an experience I had explaining my baggies of white protein powder to Jamaican customs officers in Montego Bay. While I was checking into their country to meet up with a cruise ship, they forced me to make protein smoothies for them to drink, saying they could not pass me through immigration without knowing what the powder was.

Anyway, before I knew it, my body was looking and feeling better from my high-protein, low-fat diet and the comedy career was in full swing. I soon started to notice how my healthy lifestyle set me apart from other performers. While most comedians were getting up around noon to douse last night's hangover with food, I was rising before the sun was up to work out and start the day's eating routine.

At one point, I was confronted by a comedy buddy about my, as he called it, "freakish health-nut, workout" lifestyle. He said, "You don't live like a comedy star, man! How are you ever gonna move up in this business if you don't learn how to party and tear it up a little?"

"Easy," I said. "You're all gonna die, and when I'm the only one still alive, it'll be my turn to headline." *Outlive the competition.* It wasn't much of a mantra to live by, but I'd take it.

Meanwhile on my cruise ship gigs, I found members of the ship's crews who were looking to change their bodies and their lives, and actually *wanted* my help. The struggle for people working on those ships is that food is so accessible in such great quantities, and not always very healthy. "Write me a workout," one said. "Help me with my diet!" came from others. My years of experience were about to pay off and, in turn, these amazing people were going to inspire *me*! We worked hard and, together, we made huge strides.

One of my weekly training partners, Jonathan, lost over 60 pounds, and his thirst for protein shakes was outweighed only by his thirst for knowledge. Since the day we started over 12 years ago, he's kept weight off and buffed up, and he's working towards becoming a personal trainer to help others.

My motivation was overwhelming. I had to find a way to stay in comedy *and* fitness, so I could use the latter to continue helping people make a difference in their lives. So I started hosting bodybuilding shows and writing comedy fitness articles with the goal of sneaking a bit of information in with the laughter, like when you roll your dog's medicine up in cheese so he doesn't see it coming.

That way, everything starts off all yummy and then moves to, "Aw, dammit!" Although it's not a huge dream; it's mine.

And that, along with a healthy push from my comedy mentor, was the birth of the "Fitness Comedian" and, hopefully, of a format for information that will help you make a change in *your* life.

Chapter 1

Forget What You Know

I've seen people take off their shoes, jewelry and hat, go to the bathroom, donate blood, and even shave their legs to make themselves weigh less before stepping on a scale. I don't want to think about what their legs must have looked like for shaving to have had an impact on their weigh-in, but the point is that people will do almost anything to make the needle on the scale go down. I say *almost* anything, because that "anything" usually doesn't include healthy eating. At least not what is commonly thought of as healthy.

When it comes to diet and nutrition, my experience has led me to put people in two distinctly different categories: people who say they know *exactly* what to eat but don't, and people who say they don't know what to eat or they would be in great shape. At this point, who really cares which side of that fence you're on?

It's just one big tubby game of volleyball and no one can spike.

I've also found that both groups have a wild array of pre-conceived ideas about how to "diet" when the time comes to buckle down.

Here are some of my favorites:

Switch to diet soda Forget the fact that whether we pick a diet or regular beverage, it is probably washing down a double-bacon cheeseburger and large fries. Extra soda calories *do* make a difference, but there's a bigger problem than our Big Gulp. Don't worry, though, we'll tackle your *Coke* problem later.

Don't eat after 6pm What are we, Gremlins? Don't get wet, either, or you'll multiply. (Okay, that one's true. But I don't have time to explain where babies come from.) Just know that your clock is your own. What if you work the night shift? Or what if you miss a meal and when 6 o'clock rolls around, your mind says you can't eat but your body says you need food! Don't be a clock-blocker...or a carb-blocker (Chapter 2)

I just won't eat Who needs fuel, right? Your car is lighter without all that pesky gasoline, but see how long you can drive around like that. What's next, you're going to hold your breath until the weight comes off?

This is the single biggest mistake that the vast majority of us make when it's time to shave off a few pounds.

I'll just switch to eating salads until I my weight goes down Salads, really? Some of the fattest animals on the planet are the ones that snack all day on leafy greens. And did you honestly think that taco salad was a diet food if you could eat the bowl that it came in? I can't wait for you to get to *this* chapter!

It doesn't matter what I eat, I can work it off Right, because you've been doing that for years. Every time you've eaten that extra slice of cheesecake or super-sized your lunch, you've put on your walkin' shoes and headed off. You know as well as I do, if you had really done that, you would still be on your trek, looking like one of those crazy explorers with the icicles in their beard at base-camp on Everest. The math on exercising off extra calories is outrageous: one milkshake, three-mile walk; two extra slices of pizza, two-hour swim.

The reality is that with the quality of the knowledge John or Joanne Doe has about healthy eating, they have a better chance of getting ripped while tailgating at a Jimmy Buffet concert than they do getting their body ready for beach season.

Most of this sketchy info comes from the same caliber source as the one we learned about sex from on the school playground. People hear a rumor or see something they shouldn't, and suddenly, they're experts.

From starving themselves to going on crazy diets that limit what they eat, to becoming physically ill, some people will go to any length to get the job done. The following is an actual conversation I had with a perpetually dieting friend.

Me: "Wow, what a rough weekend! I had food poisoning and lost eight pounds."

Friend: "Eight pounds in a weekend, what did you eat?"

Me: "I got hold of some bad scallops at Randy's Grill."

Friend: "Wow! Do you think they have any left?"

Me: "What do you mean?"

Friend: "That's really awesome, losing eight pounds in a couple days. I've got a wedding to go to this Saturday. I'd better get down to Randy's before they throw out the rest of the scallops!"

So where *do* you get information you can trust? The place that you are supposed to learn about getting in shape the right way is one that cracks me up the most: "Consult your physician." Sure, I'll drive down to the medical center, walk through the group of nurses smoking on their break and ask my out-of-shape doctor for his insights. I'm sure a guy who thinks running errands and jogging his memory counts as exercise will be a fountain of knowledge.

Whether you think the Red Hot Chili Peppers and the Black-Eyed Peas are "food groups" or that the Food Pyramid is a multi-level marketing scheme doesn't matter. Whatever you believe is the key to losing weight and getting toned or ripped, forget it! The healthiest thing you could have at this point is a clean "plate" for new information.

Dear Diary

One of the first things I do with anyone I try to help lose weight is have them write down everything they eat for three days. And I mean *everything*! That includes every meal and snack, every swoop they make past the office candy dish like an eagle plucking a trout from a stream (or, if you live in a big city, like someone picking your pocket on the subway), and especially everything they drink.

Most people just ask me to write down what *I* think they should eat. This is usually followed by, "Are you serious? That sounds nasty! I want to lose a few pounds, not go to Survivor Island."

By writing down (or entering into your fancy i-Thing) everything you eat and drink, you can see where you could make changes towards dropping a few easy lbs. The biggest challenge outside of being thorough is not to treat your food diary like one of those "Are you an honest person?" quizzes in a magazine where you try to answer the right way so you come across as a wonderful person. Lying on the honesty test gets you nowhere. And, FYI, finishing the "Are you great in bed quiz?" really fast apparently makes you lose 10 points.

The best way to keep a food diary is to keeping a running tab all day like a to-do list, so you don't forget things. It will probably be more like a "to-don't" list, but ignore that and just jot down whenever you eat or drink *anything*. Add the times too; we'll cover the importance of that in a minute. Your list may appear to be a depressing daily recap that makes Anne Frank's diary seem like letters sent home from summer camp, but at least it will be accurate. For an example of what I'm talking about, check out this re-creation with details from the diary of someone I worked with a few years ago:

"Dear Diary, Damn, can I put away the food! My day started with a dream that I was a contestant on 'Jeopardy' and in my sleep I smacked the snooze button a few extra times to give Alex Trebek the answers. Needless to say, I missed my shot at making breakfast so I stopped off at the coffee place for an Iced Mocha Frappe with whipped cream and cookie chunks, and in order to eat healthy, I grabbed a bran muffin.

Four hours later, I was famished and it was Stacy from HR's birthday. She got to pick the lunch place, and chose one of those family-style Italian restaurants. I don't know how big her family is, but the 'style' was food on plates the size of hubcaps. It was delish, but I needed a little nap at my desk after lunch. Good thing I wore my stretchy pants today.

I still felt full when I got home and also felt guilty, so I skipped dinner. Well, sort of. I had a glass of wine, then another, and got hungry. I know it was 10 o'clock at night, but it's better to eat than skip meals, right? I didn't have the energy to cook and thankfully had some leftover Thai from the other night. I think it was still good; Thai smells funky when it's fresh. It was spicy, so I had one more glass of wine.

Oh, and I forgot, we split a couple pitchers of Sangria at lunch and shared a dessert. Ugh! Maybe the leftovers will be bad and I'll get sick and lose what I ate today. If not, I guess I'll walk it off."

Your journal doesn't have to be that detailed or dramatic. It could be as simple as:

7:30 am 2 Sausage McMuffins and a large coffee

10:00 am Chunk of donut from break room, more coffee

12:0 pm Caesar Salad with Salmon, 2 breadsticks, large Coke

1:30 pm can of coke

6:00 pm Healthy Choice Lasagna dinner, 1 glass Red Wine

9:30 pm Chips and Dip, 1 more glass Red Wine

By looking back at that day's eating journal and reading the next few chapters, you should be able to diagnose where you can shave off a few hundred calories a day without feeling like a diet hostage. You might be shocked at how just taking off a little bit every day will lead to big results over the long haul. One pound here and half a pound there will have weight falling off faster than Justin Beiber's career after his voice changed.

Stop starving yourself!

In an effort to lose a few pounds, have you ever decided to just skip a few meals, but by the end of the day you were gnawing on a table leg? Ever wonder why the first demand of shooters holed-up in a clock tower is a pizza? Skipping meals causes your blood sugar to drop and your body's chemical reaction is to say, "I don't give a shit about your diet; I want food now!"

To calm the savage beast, your body will probably crave high-carbohydrate (high sugar) food to feed its need for insulin, which totally screws up exactly what you were trying to accomplish. And when your blood sugar drops, so does your judgment. By avoiding food to lose weight, you are using the same level of thought the average teenager uses when they say, "How could this possibly go wrong?"

Skipping meals is probably the number ONE thing that people do when they want to lose weight. After all, if what caused us to gain a few extra pounds was eating too much, then the obvious answer is to eat less. If that's true, then the best way to lose it even faster is to stop eating altogether, right? Whether you want to believe this or not, that is the *worst* thing you can do!

I'm not sure why they call not eating "fasting," because it immediately slows your metabolism down and puts your body into hibernation. And what's the first thing we think of when we hear the word "hibernation," a bear of course! And yet bears don't have a body shape we want. Have you ever seen the ass on a black bear? I'm just saying. Most bears have the majority of their weight in the lower half, a look that is totally "grizzly" to most of us. Actually, polar bears are the largest in the species, but have smaller butts because they tend to do Pilates and stay away from fried foods.

Unlike what occurs with a bear, though, your food hibernation doesn't necessarily tap into your fat stores for energy. This is because often, the easiest thing for your body to eat is muscle. The result is the look called "skinny fat" in dieters, one in which your body is lighter but still manages to look flabby and less healthy.

Spiders can also go long periods without eating, and look at their shapes. If we could hear spider conversations, they would probably sound like:

"You know, ever since I had those last few thousand babies, I just can't seem to get my thorax back."

"I know what you're saying, Margie. My new husband made a wisecrack about how the web was sagging under my weight, and I bit his head off."

I mentioned the word metabolism, which in this case basically means the speed in which your body breaks down food for energy. Even more specifically, the unit of energy created from the breakdown of food in the form of "body heat" is called a calorie. (See, Mr. Headley, I *was* listening. I just hated homework.)

Let's break this down even more. When you process food for energy (digestion) you create heat in the body, so think of your metabolism like a campfire. When you want a fire to rage you add kindling, usually little sticks and twigs. In the world of diet, this kindling is those small, frequent meals you hear so much about. If you skip a meal, or two, then have a big meal, it is the equivalent of letting your fire die down almost completely and then throwing a big log on it. If that doesn't make the fire go out, it will definitely take a lot longer to get it going again and the log will be one that burns unevenly. When your fire inside dies down and burns food unevenly, this is one of the ways your body stores food as fat.

By the way, if all of this talk about campfires is making you think about S'mores, then we have a bigger issue than a quick lesson on frequent meals. So get back to business.

The other important point here is that while eating up to 3-4 small meals a day would be great (or at least two or three with healthy snacks in between), the quality of those meals is equally as important. A calorie is NOT a calorie. For a more obvious example; a grilled chicken breast, brown rice, and steamed veggie plate that contains 450 calories is not nutritionally equal to a king-sized Snickers bar. I know, you're probably saying, "Well duh!" But if that was obvious to everyone, I wouldn't be pointing it out.

As a matter of fact, let's even reinforce that a bit more. Let's get back to your car for a minute. If your gas tank holds 15 gallons, you put in 15 gallons of *gasoline,* not vinegar and water. If you've ever heard your engine knock like you had someone trapped under the hood then you know the quality of gas makes a difference, too. So, don't be a douche; put good food in your tank.

I had a personal training client a long time ago for whom I had written out an extremely detailed diet. But she kept asking how many calories she should be eating every day.

After a few weeks of her body not making any positive progress, and actually going backwards a bit, I had to ask, "Are you following the eating plan I gave you?"

"Sort of," she said. "I'm eating the number calories you suggested. I just modified the plan a bit to suit my liking."

"Modified how?" inquiring minds wanted to know.

"Well, you said I could have 1,600 calories a day. So I figured if I didn't eat for a day, then on the second day I could have a medium pizza with everything, right? Eight slices is about 3,200 calories."

She was not even close. I eventually had to stop training her because her dad was paying me and he was *huge*. No way was I going to let her lack of dietary discipline cost me my life!

The takeaway here is that to get your metabolic fire really burning, you should start first thing in the morning with a small, healthy breakfast (Protein, carbs, fruits and vegetables) and keep adding a little bit of quality food all day. While everyone's body is a little different, the magic number that seems to work for most people is eating every three or four hours. If you find that doesn't work for your schedule, try to plan your healthy snacks to cover the gaps in between.

Don't miss meals if you can avoid it. But if you do, don't try to make up for the missing calories or give in to your body screaming for junk food.

Instead, drink a full glass of water as soon as you sit down to eat, and wait a few minutes for that to fill you up.

Another thing for your diet that can be a bigger trip-up than a man walking around wearing high heels is trying to add too many meals or making too many healthy changes at once. If you currently eat once or maybe twice a day, then suddenly overwhelming yourself with all of the cooking, eating, and going to the bathroom that comes with a healthier lifestyle is dooming your diet to failure.

Instead, start by adding one snack to your day's intake. It doesn't have to be anything fancy; maybe try yogurt, fruit, nuts, veggies, and a low-fat dip, basically anything that doesn't come out of a vending machine or a package. A good rule is if a food can stay "alive" inside of a machine, it's probably causing death inside of human.

Build up to eating healthy. What you are starting is a better relationship with food, so it's probably not a good idea to go all the way with your diet on the first date. And don't make the next mistake, spending night and day with chicken and broccoli for a few weeks until you get sick of it. Before you know it, the new and exciting changes you made to your eating plan wear off and you start noticing all the things that annoy you.

Soon, you can't stand the way it smells or looks and you don't know how to find moderation, so you just ignore it and stop calling. Worse yet, you cheat on it with some dirty pizza late at night, only to feel guilty in the morning when you see the box. You shamefully walk it out to the trash in the morning and hope no one sees you. It's too much to bear!

 Go easy. You and your new healthy lifestyle have your whole lives together, so take your time.

I'll just have a salad

This is the official battle cry of wanna-be dieters everywhere. The reality is that you stand a better chance of making a dent in your flab by falling asleep on the remote control than you do turning to salads. This idea has all of the planning, forethought, and probable success of a blind-folded whack at a piñata. The difference, of course, is if little Brittany or Zachary (or insert another overplayed GenX baby's name here) actually connects with the Dora the Explorer effigy, they have real candy to look forward to.

The salad-eater, however, knows that their prize is usually nothing more than a pile of wet leaves drenched in fat. Let's face it; if it wasn't for a little Ranch dressing, the average salad would look and taste like something we pluck off of our shoes before going indoors.

I don't know where the salad craze started or what we really think we're going to accomplish by grazing on a plate of moist greens. But let's take a few minutes to pick apart the reality of losing weight eating the sacred salad.

First, I would be doing you a great disservice if I didn't start with the most basic facts, the nutritional value of lettuce. Depending on where you get your information, you will wind up with a variety of answers. If you ask at your local health food store, someone who hasn't shaved or bathed in a while may break away from a conversation about saving an indigenous people from the evils of cell phones to tell you how amazing salads are. That is, of course, if Moonbeam's iron-deficient, energy-drained, vegan body can reach you for this lesson on the power of greens.

"I eat them, juice with them, and even use them as toilet paper and rub them under my pits for deodorant," they might say. They may even drive their point home by saying lettuce is packed with vitamins, minerals, protein, fiber, and more.

I laughed and threw up in my mouth while typing that, by the way, as it is a plate-load of hooey. Iceberg lettuce, which is

what makes up most restaurant salads, has trace amounts of protein and fiber (1g or less), and maybe if you're lucky, a little vitamin K which is important for helping your blood to clot. This may turn out be a bad thing after your arteries close up from the cheese and dressing you end up using to give your pile of lettuce any flavor. For the sake of remembering this, think of your diet as the Titanic and your salad, well, that's the iceberg.

So what is the truth behind the leaves? The truth is that most varieties of lettuce seem to be missing enough nutrition by themselves to be food. Friends, Romaines, and countrymen, lend me your Butterleafs. It turns out that romaine lettuce is missing almost any value. Yes, it's low in sodium and calories (almost zero), but wet paper can say the same.

Before you think about making a snack out of paper, however, it's important that you know I'm talking about notebook paper, as the average newspaper today has no value, nutritional or informational. Meanwhile, back in the produce section, at least Butterleaf, Bibb lettuce, and especially spinach, have *some* nutrients. So *head* in that direction, just not too fast. There's more…

If I haven't turned the warning sign around from Slow to STOP for you yet, let's go a little further…

Tim Wilkins

When you eat a salad, do you ever order just a plate of lettuce? No, you get something with a fancy name, like Caesar, Chef, or Wedge Salad.

Figuring out this part couldn't be any easier; just look at the names and they speak for themselves. Caesar, a salad named after an obese Roman emperor. Pass! As for the Chef salad, that's an odd name for something that took almost no cooking. And when was the last time you saw a thin chef?

The "wedgie" is, of course, what you get when your underwear goes in your butt, which coincidentally seems to happen more frequently as you get out of shape. But I guess that makes sense, as a Wedge salad is nothing more than a triangle of iceberg lettuce coated in a large amount of bacon and fatty sauce which will eventually end up on your backside. Get ready to start digging out your underpants.

According to my heroes who write the "*Eat This, Not That!*" series of books, there are actually 20 salads in restaurants that are nutritionally worse

42

than a Whopper. Knowing that, who in their right mind wouldn't want the Whopper instead? As always in their books, there are healthier alternatives given to each of the gut-bombs listed in their top 20 list. But to give you an idea of what you're up against by eating salads as diet food:

16. Fiesta Taco Salad (Taco Bell) This fiesta is no party at 770 calories and 42g of fat. Rule of thumb is if you can eat the bowl, it's probably bad for you.

This goes for soups served in giant bread vats, too.

12. Applebee's Shrimp and Spinach Salad (Um, Applebee's. Apples are healthy and bees make honey, so it must be good for you.) Shrimp? Spinach? How could this be wrong? Well, it actually has 1070 calories and 69g of fat and we haven't even broken the Top 10 yet.

Of course, there's Chili's Quesadilla Explosion Salad. (Using the magic of looking at the key words in food, do you want to eat anything called "explosion"?)

And then we move on to the number 1 worst salad in the land, according to "*ETNT*" guru David Zinczenko. This would be TGI Friday's Santa Fe Chopped Salad. Not since banditos roamed New Mexico, has anyone stood the chance of being treated this badly in Santa Fe. At a whopping 1830 calories, this salad would give you a full day's worth of intake, yet only one-fourth of the valuable nutrients your body needs.

So what makes salad a good part of your healthy food plan? The secret is what you do, or don't, put on it. Lettuce itself being nearly worthless makes it only a delightful foundation to put your *food* on. (They call it a *bed* of lettuce for a reason.) All you filthy-minded types can go ahead and get excited by this next part: let your greens be a good place to put your meat. (I heard sex sells, and if it means you will eat better, expect this tactic again throughout the book.)

Pack your salad with lean proteins like meat, chicken, fish, and eggs. Be sure to order or make those proteins grilled, blackened, or baked, and not breaded and fried, which totally defeats the purpose.

Top that off with a wide variety of fruits or vegetables that have a lot of vitamins and minerals *and* dietary fiber. Beans, or as the fancy people call them, "legumes," are excellent things to throw on top of your salad to increase your protein and fiber at the same time.

If we are starting at ground zero with your fitness knowledge, no worries; I'm talking about chickpeas (garbanzos), cannellini beans, kidney beans, pintos, and more. You may need a little Bean-O to help keep your relationships alive when you increase your legume intake, but whatever it takes, right? Besides, if you're looking hot and feeling good about yourself, you'll be sexy enough to overcome the fact that you've turned into a gas factory.

That leaves only the "what *not*" to put on it. Where we go terribly wrong with having "just a salad" is throwing fatty cheese, bacon, and dressing all over the top of it. These toppings make the average salad a high-calorie food, not to mention that it is bursting with salt and saturated fat.

Of course, the favorite dressing for many people is Ranch. And we know what lives on a ranch…pigs and cows! Ranch dressing, even the low-fat version, is 80%, yes, 80%, fat!

Most dressings are made with oils that are high in fat, the store-bought kinds are not quality oil, and when we do apply dressings we don't exactly spray them on with a fine mist of flavor do we? A little spritz? Aw, hell no! Spritzes are only done by evil-looking perfume counter ladies with white coats and eyebrows painted on to make them appear shocked by the world. Salad dressing is usually slopped on using a ladle and all the same care and concern as the lunchroom lady used to dump food on our tray in school. So we offset any possible goodness that could come from our salad by burying it under a sea of cholesterol-laden goop. Oh, make no mistake, it's tasty. But you won't look or feel any better after eating it, and it definitely is *not* diet food.

When it comes time to add your dressing, think about just that, dressing…or rather, undressing. Knowing full well that any sauces you use are going to end up being seen on your body, do you want your body to be something heavy and goopy or something light? Of course, you want something light, so a bit of oil and vinegar, herbs, pepper, lemon, or a low-fat and low-sodium dressing is the way to go.

If you end up grazing at a salad bar, stay away from fatty sides like potato salad and coleslaw, as they are loaded with high-fat mayonnaise. Also, avoid toppings like nuts, bacon, and croutons.

Salad can be a nutritional minefield, so step lightly!

Are you going to eat *all* of that?

When it comes to how *much* to eat in order to lose weight or live a healthy lifestyle, proper food portions can be so hard to understand. A lot of diets give us catchy food quantities created to make things more understandable.

Ten grams of this, 25 grams of that; the only ones who know the metric system are scientists and people who have done drugs. I guess that explains why members of both groups are usually skinny.

Maybe using those terms would be the key to connecting with more people. Okay, here goes: your protein portion should be the size of a nickel bag, an 8-Ball of fat, and at least half a kilo of fruits and vegetables per day.

And then there are the quantities designed for degenerate gamblers: your protein should be the size of a deck of cards, fats the size of dice, and fruit and vegetable portions should look like two stacks of $100 chips.

That's an odd reference, considering that casinos are known for giving away tickets to buffets and not weekend makeovers with a personal trainer. In a casino, there is only going to be one "Biggest Loser."

While I don't want to over-stress that it is quantity or quality that makes the difference in weight loss, if you had to start somewhere, let it be with how much you are eating. If we could possibly eat just a little bit of the things we enjoy, instead of enough to feed a small village, we would stand a much better chance of staying healthy... and hot.

Of course, restraint would be a nifty tool to utilize if we had it, but none of us seems to have any these days. And the only thing that seems to be getting smaller in the world is not our portion sizes but our cell phones.

This really sucks, because as phones shrink to the size of a TicTac, they are harder to hold with our pudgier fingers.

Food manufacturers are *not* helping us, as some of the "muffin top" we are developing is due to the fact that our breakfast muffins look more like birthday cakes. One study showed muffins to be almost 333% bigger than the portion standards set by the USDA. And the average bagel is bigger than most of the hokey spare tires that now come with new cars. So, thanks to both bigger bread products and smaller spares, we now have "junk" in our trunks.

Gone should be the days when putting away two pancakes the size of Frisbees is acceptable, especially when they are topped with a Rubik's Cube-size "pat" of butter. No bigger than a CD should be the size rule for pancakes. Otherwise, after eating a serving or two a week, you will quickly go from IHOP to I waddle.

And forget bellying up to that bowl of pasta the size of Saint Bernard's food dish. It's really not doing you any favors. The average bowl of noodles at your favorite restaurant (or at the home of your obese Aunt Marie who insists you're skinny), is approximately 500% bigger than this carbohydrate portion should be. Cut back on the noodles and add a bit more sauce and maybe a veggie or two. Primavera, anyone?

All-you-can-eat buffets are all the rage, and for some sad reason we have turned them into a personal challenge. We mosey in, walk the hot lines, and put more thought into our eating attack than we do into our retirement planning. From there, you and the waitress get in a stare-down that would rival the standoff at the OK Corral. The only difference is that you're not a gunslinger.

You're on the other side of the corral fence, about to run squealing up to the feed trough like prize livestock. The men tend to go for the meat, the women for the salad bar, and the kids for the pizza and ice cream; sometimes for the ice cream pizza. When the carnage is over, pants are unbuttoned and the war begins to see who can push the table farthest away from their side of the booth. Oink!

Unless you are trying to survive on one meal for a few days or prepping for a trip to the electric chair, there is no good reason to eat that much in one sitting.

And heaven forbid it's one of those Brazilian steak places where they walk around with meat on a sword.

I went to one with a friend who turned it into an eating challenge bigger than the rap battle in the movie "*8 Mile*."

Tim Wilkins

One more way we are sabotaged is the stupid things that manufacturers do when they try to make it "easy" for those of us attempting to maintain our weight, like portioning things out in 100-calorie snack packs. Great! Now we have to eat eight of them to be full. There goes five bucks, and we still ate the same amount of junk food. At least we burned some energy opening the packages.

We even have marketers telling us how we can stay on track through the glory of the Tic Tac, which has only five calories. Really? Shouldn't anything be that low in calories you need tweezers to eat? And was that candy, or did I just swallow my cell phone?

In many ways, the tables, and plates, are literally stacked against us. Two ways to ace the average AYCE buffet are to drink a big glass of water as soon as you sit down and to eat slowly. By doing this, you both fill your stomach a bit with the water and start signaling your body with the chemicals that tell it you have had enough to eat. (Just wondering what the world's population

52

would be if our bodies had a chemical to tell us that we've had enough alcohol?)

FYI, these chemicals that tell us when we are full take a few minutes to kick in. Until then, ease off the throttle a bit, Maverick.

As for how much to eat at home or away, the palm of your hand is a good protein size for meat, chicken, and fish. It's true what they say, small hands, small feet, small meat...requirements. Fibers and fruits (this includes pasta, potatoes, and starchy vegetables like broccoli and asparagus) should be no bigger than your tightly clinched fist. If you want to lose weight, use the hands of someone smaller. Get it? Palm=Protein, Fist=Fibers and Fruits, for Fats...it's another F, finger.

(As in give them the middle finger!) Eat good fats like nuts, healthy oils, and avocado in portions about the size of your thumb at every meal. Bad fats like butter and oil are another digit, however; the middle finger.

Chapter 2

Don't Believe What You See or Hear, Either

In 1989, Robert Fulghum released the book, "*All I Really Need to Know I Learned in Kindergarten.*" While the premise and the writing were great, I don't think taking naps, making macaroni necklaces, and remembering not to pee your pants is enough advice to get people through the next 50 to 80 years. This is especially true when it comes to nutrition.

When we were in kindergarten, snacks were provided which usually consisted of either a PB&J sandwich or chocolate milk. Nowadays, we know that some kids have a nut allergy, some are lactose intolerant, and there may even be a kid or two who is both. Just look for the ones having seizures in a cloud of gas, hold your nose and stick them with epi-pens as needed.

Today, the average kindergartner lives on chicken nuggets and juice boxes, and gets a toy as a reward for eating them. The K and pre-K years aside, we are taught *almost* enough by sixth grade to actually live a healthy life. We are shown the food pyramid and the food groups, and given a thorough lesson (or ten) about junk food.

Unfortunately, however, when the bell rings after those classes, we dash off to the cafeteria for Nacho Tuesday.

This begs the question that if we pretty much know what healthy eating is, then why do we fall for all of the hype and BS the diet world feeds us? It seems the fine line between common sense and free will is drawn using bread sticks and churros, and while we may know what we *should* be eating, we simply chose not to.

When asked what is part of a healthy eating regimen or what are the right things to eat to lose weight, most people freeze up with the same dopey look on their face they had when the bouncer asked them whose picture was on their fake ID. I usually combat this bit of selective memory with a pop quiz you can take here:

Question 1:

If you had to choose between two beverages, which is more healthy:

a)   8 oz. of water

or

b)   8 oz. of bacon fat

(Hint: Unless it's still hot, bacon fat isn't very liquid.)

Question 2:

You have only two possibilities for breakfast. Do you eat:

a)   The raspberry Pop-Tarts that say they are made with real "fruit"

or

b)   An egg sandwich on whole grain bread

The answers to those questions are always quick and correct, and I am met with a "What do you think I am, an idiot?" expression. This proves pretty quickly that the client in question does indeed know what they *should* be eating. And so do you. For the record, those are not really very extreme examples; they are actually very similar to the choices we are faced with almost every time we eat.

So if that's not an issue, what is it? From what I can see, we use our free will to choose what we want to believe.

To make matters worse, there is never any shortage of items to pick from when it comes to justifying our eating habits. On the contrary, it seems more like a case of another major issue: TMI (too much information).

TMI is like when our parents tell us they had a "fun" vacation. Without details, our minds race as we consider the exciting times they had, but we're not quite sure we believe that they had a good time. But when they tell us they had great dinners and saw beautiful sights, we believe their stories and our thoughts calm down.

However, if they go on to tell us what happened in the hotel room after that second bottle of Pinot Grigio, we have achieved TMI, and all previous knowledge is pushed out of our brains to protect us. Instant information overload.

That is basically what happens every time we open a magazine or a newspaper or turn on the TV. There is a constant flow of media vomit that has our heads spinning faster than our bedroom does after a Cinco de Mayo tequila binge.

It seems like every day, some new study is released about what was bad for us is now good and what was good is now bad. We are then deluged with the details of that story, which has been triple-checked by Dr. Heywood Jablowme, MD, PhD, BFD. The realities of the study are usually in microscopic print that detail who funded the research, how many people were in the study group, and what the rest of their lives looked like in the way of healthy habits. None of that really matters, anyway, as all of the study is quickly overlooked by somebody's mom who calls their aunt who then tells her kids the newly formed gospel.

"I saw it on that doctor show," says Aunt Louise. "You know, the one where they talk about poop all the time. It must be true!" Then she goes on to say, "Without enough calcium, your bones will bend and leave you shaped like a Hobbit. And did I tell you milk is bad for you, so we should get calcium from beans and greens?"

Yeah, *that's* gonna happen. So find a bowl, kids, because from now on, we're gonna score our RDA of calcium from kale and chickpeas.

The confusion in this area goes on and on. Coffee is good for you; no, wait; it's bad. Fat is bad for your unless it's *good* fat and then, of course, it's great for you.

There's always a creative way to feel better about ourselves, so maybe it would help us all emotionally not to say we're obese, we're just *good* fat. That isn't a fat roll over my belt; it's a stockpile of Omega-3 fatty acids.

And what the hell is gluten and how have I survived this long eating so much of it? The butt muscle is called the "glute," so if eating gluten is giving me a fatty ass, get it out of my food.

If you've ever tried to buy products that are gluten-free, you know they are the anything but "free." Why are we forking over some much cash for gluten removal?

The food pyramid has been the ultimate multi-level marketing scheme. It appears now that it was collaboration between the government and the food producers to try to sell bigger harvests. If there was a bumper crop of corn and wheat, the "pyramid" was changed to tell us we needed a few more servings of grains. Our current President has changed the shape of the pyramid to round; and, yes, that is pie-shaped! When called on the carpet about that, however, the Obama Administration said it was shaped more like, I kid you not, a veggie pizza.

Alcohol drinking recommendations have changed over the years from suggesting one glass of red wine per day for optimum heart health to two. Now, however, it is up to two drinks of *any* kind. Before you know it, the liquor lobby will commission a study saying that the perfect amount per day is four or more drinks. So in order to have a long and happy life, most of us will need to live in the gutter. I guess if you think about it, we all have those relatives we thought should have died years ago, but are actually pickled in booze. Ah, what to believe…

And then there is the endless supply of stories about how to change your body instantly: "Flatten your butt while sitting" and "Burn fat while you sleep." "Get Clooney's abs" or "Madonna's shredded shoulders." Short of gaining these ideal *parts* by abducting our favorite celebs, the reality of how to get them isn't in the three-page article. These stars have personal trainers, personal chefs, and someone who personally airbrushes away their "imperfections." Not to mention that if they have kids, they have someone to take care of them so the stars have all that extra time to work out and look fab.

And FYI, guys, if your significant other ever says, "I'd sure like to have Demi Moore or Cameron Diaz's body," do not under *any* circumstances say, "Me, too!"

Speaking of which, I love the scene in "*Something About Mary*" in which Ben Stiller is in the car with a crazed Harland Williams who is telling him about his new workout program, "*6-Minute Abs*." The blowout begins when Ben asks, "What happens when someone comes along with "*5-Minute Abs*?" To which Harland screams the reply, "You can't do abs in five minutes!"

We know there really are no magic workout moves that will give us rocking bodies overnight without hard work, but we want so badly to believe there are. Fitness can be like Santa; the day you stop believing is the day the giant haul of gifts becomes just one crappy present with a tag that reads, "From Mom and Dad." So how do you work your way through the muddled puddle of fitness and diet myths?

First, stop believing everything you see and hear. The surest way to be out of shape is to swallow all of the make-believe hype we are fed by the media to sell stuff. When it comes to what to eat, try wading through the constant flow of gossip and well-funded BS by taking everything with, well, a grain of salt. (Unless you have high blood pressure, of course. Please consult your physician before adding any rhetorical grains of salt to your psyche.)

I'll say it throughout the book: you know what to eat. It's all about balance, moderation, and whole, unprocessed foods like meat, grains, fruits, and vegetables. It really is that simple; if it can go bad, it's good for you. If it can't, it isn't.

When it comes to working out, there is one perfect, secret *move* I've never read about in any magazine. The best motion to tighten your whole body, abs, butt, etc., is called the "Push Away." That means push away your plate when you are full, and never continue eating just because food is in front of you.

Push away from the mindless eating in the car or in front of your TV or computer. And when it comes to exercise, an unhappy marriage is the perfect home gym. When you push away your spouse at night, use your arms one night and your legs the next, always keeping your stomach tight. As he or she gains weight, you get stronger. See? There's a positive side to everything!

TV chefs are trying to kill us

I have to start off by saying that I have loved cooking and watching people cook on TV since I was a teenager. From Martin Yan to the self-marinating Cajun, Justin Wilson, I have long been enthralled by TV "chefery." Back then, however, watching someone cook on TV wasn't quite such a hip thing for people to do, especially not young boys. I'm not saying that I wasn't cool, but I didn't exactly want to admit that while the popular kids were watching "CHiPs" and "Battlestar Galactica," I was watching an English chef make a Beef Wellington.

Recently, however, cooking on the small screen took on a new life when shows did the same thing that the country music industry did to suck us in, by making the chefs hotter or more like family members.

They even added the American spirit of competition, pitting chef against chef at every turn.

What they won't tell you about this programming plot is that it's trying to kill you! I'm generally not a conspiracy theorist, but I'm convinced that more than a couple of the culinary rock stars want us dead! We may not have met, and I really don't know what we did to provoke them, but there are a few in particular that I believe have it in for us.

One is a raspy little Smurfette who whips up recipes with an unhealthy blend of cute and Mafia. In less than 30 minutes, she creates a Sammy you can't refuse, and therein lies the problem. She's so entertaining, so likeable, that we manage to overlook the fact that so much of what she makes is just not good for us. Oh, it might taste

"Yummo," but if you can break away from her hypnotic dimples and shot glasses of EVOO long enough to think about a bacon, cheese, and prosciutto sandwich on buttered cheese bread, you might want to switch channels to a home shopping network and pick up some defib paddles.

Then there's another one who couldn't look and sound any more like my favorite aunt if she crawled out of a cloning machine. It's not even fair to put her on TV without Hug-O-Vision! Everything she cooks reminds me of that side of my family, too. From the fresh baked biscuits and gravy we used to consume before fishing trips, and the pies and cakes that were to die for...literally.

I've actually heard her joke about "delicious death" in the recipes more than once. On one episode, she mentioned that she was starting the recipe with two sticks of butter, asking with a smile, "Did Y'all think there was any other way I would start out?" She followed that up with a cup of sugar and blended in a cup of whole cream.

Even the Cuisinart had a hard time processing it, so imagine what your arteries would go through.

That said, it came as no big shock when this Queen of Southern Cuisine broke the news that she has Type 2 Diabetes. In the immortal words of another Southern star, Gomer Pyle, "Sur-prise, Sur-prise, Sur-prise!" Do you mean to tell me that someone who puts butter on blocks of fried Velveeta is in poor health?

She didn't fool *me* with her sweet smile and her chili cheese fries, but, sadly, she roped in a couple million other people who followed her recipe for bad health. Fortunately, she won't continue to lead people to their doom (even though she apparently did for three years while waiting to tell us about her health problems), because she is turning over a new spatula.

Always one to turn lemons into lemon chiffon pie, that special someone has traded her sponsorship deal with Land O' Lakes for one with a new diabetes medication named Victoza that apparently can be injected with a turkey baster.

Other than the fact that she's a savvy marketer, what's the lesson from this that we should put in the to-go box? Here are several:

Just because it's on TV doesn't mean it's good for you. Case in point, "Jersey Shore." It may seem like fun at first, but being drunk and orange is not a good long-term life plan.

- Just because it tastes good does not mean it is good for you. As a matter of fact, just the opposite.

    Much of the "drugs" in Southern food, (fat, sugar, and salt) are things our bodies have become addicted to and now crave. We need to break our dependency and train ourselves to enjoy natural flavors. Which leads me to my final point...

- Have I mentioned moderation yet? Butter, cheese, meat, and even foods that are good for you can become bad for you in large amounts.

If you've ever been to a buffet and been "cut off," then you know where I'm going. Eating a little bit of everything could go a long way toward keeping you healthy.

The next time you're watching your favorite chefs on TV, enjoy the way their dishes look, enjoy their flair for the dramatic when they scream "Bam!" or when they eat a giant, cheese-stuffed hot pepper like only a hipster with sunglasses on backwards can, but think twice before you try to recreate, much less eat, what they make.

Chapter 3

Take it Off *Really* Slow

So you've put on a couple of pounds, huh? Did the "freshman 10" turn in to the post-graduate 20 or 30? Maybe you had a baby and couldn't shed the weight, or your wife got pregnant and because you're such a great guy, you put on 40 "sympathy" pounds. The sad part for you is that most of her weight fell off when the baby came, but you couldn't breastfeed to get rid of your new man boobs, or "moobs," as they're called.

Or maybe you just got caught up in life and while you were busy trying to get ahead, you put on a few extra pounds in your behind? Whatever the cause, now you're looking in the mirror or down at the scale and you want to do something about what you see. So what *do* you do? Go on a diet, right? WRONG! Going *on* a diet is where we go wrong. A diet isn't something you go on. Saying you're going "on" something means that you only plan to do it for a short time, like "I'm going *on* a bike ride" or "I'm going *on* a trip," acid or otherwise.

Saying you're going *on* a diet is the same as going *on* a rollercoaster. Your weight will go up and down, you'll scream a little, maybe throw up, and then end up right back where you started. And in both cases, you will probably be thinking, "Stop this thing, I wanna get off!" Well, go ahead and stop. Stop dieting and stop torturing yourself with bouts of starvation and the emotional abuse of failure. Seriously, screw it, go get a piece of pizza and relax.

If you are smart, which you obviously are, then you not only want to look better but you also want to live a longer and fuller life. To accomplish this, there will be no more going *on* a diet for you. You will have to change the way you eat... forever! (Insert evil laugh here: "Muah ha ha!")

I know you're thinking, "There is no way I'm going to stop eating pizza, cheeseburgers, fries, desserts or even those deep-fried cubes of butter at the state fair." I wouldn't dare take any of that away from you, for fear of being bumped off. Somebody reading this could tell the fast-food Mafia, and there would be a "sit-down." A big table with all the families would meet in a warehouse and the Colonel, the King, Ronald, Wendy, and Tim Horton (shout-out to Canada), would all be there. A "to-go" order would be put out and they'd find me bludgeoned to death with a Happy Meal toy in an incident made to look like an accident.

With this new way of eating I'm suggesting, you can still have junk food, but, like a Smurf with his pants pulled down, "Once in a blue moon!" That will be the big switch in your life. You will *have* a diet, not be *on* a diet. A diet is, according to the Merriam-Webster's Dictionary (Yes, the online one. I'm not that friggin' old!):

Noun: The kinds of food that a person, animal, or community habitually eats.

The key word in that sentence is not "animal," although I've seen my share of people whose diets make them look like hyenas taking down a wildebeest on the Discovery Channel. The important word here is "habitually."

In order for you to achieve the look and feel you want, eating right can't be a temporary way of life until you hit your goal weight, or until your blood pressure goes back down from what the doctor called, "higher than Charlie Sheen on a webcam." Making good food choices will have to be something you think about the majority of the time when you eat, until it becomes so second-nature that you don't notice you're no longer thinking about it.

Again, your mind is screaming, "I want to lose the weight NOW!" Riiight. And I wanted a monkey with a diaper for a pet after watching "BJ and the Bear," but that didn't happen. For the record, we don't always think about the repercussions of our immediate wants. Since that early dream, what I have learned is that monkeys stink and they bite, and *I* would have had to change that diaper.

Then how will you shed those unwanted pounds? The way you are going to do it this time is by *not* falling for the latest get-thin-quick scheme. You will lose weight in the most healthy and long-lasting way possible: by changing your eating habits a little bit over time. I know, I know, it sounds really boring and too good to be true. But stay with the tour, please.

Tattoos, piercings, and fad diets

At various points throughout our lives, trends come around that define each generation. Thankfully though, except for the pictures of you looking like Madonna, MC Hammer, or part of a Flock of Seagulls, in most cases there will be no physical evidence that you were ever sucked into a particular fad.

Other trends, like tattoos, however, leave a permanent mark that may not look or feel as good as the years roll on. For example: Although it seemed like a great idea on that drunken getaway to Cancun to have the sun and the moon tattooed on your chest, after a few years of sagging, they will be a lot less sexy, and your cleavage will look more like a partial eclipse.

Another fad that could have an impact in the form of damage to your body is the fad diet. Interestingly, a lot of these diet trends come in and go out of fashion, like bell bottoms, plaid, and hair styles that make you look like you just woke up.

Think about the words "fad" and "diet" for a minute. Does either one of them by itself sound like anything worth doing? Fads don't last; but if they did, heaven help us all, right?

People will do anything to drop unwanted weight and, like anything else nowadays, they'd like to do it as quickly and effortlessly as possible. We seem to think that by focusing on one food or one food group, we can trick our bodies into somehow losing overnight the weight from the pizza we've been eating 3 days a week for 15 years. We think that if we follow the cleanse diet of drinking warm water with maple syrup and cayenne pepper, we can flush out a lifetime of bad food choices and instantly snap into shape. I can save you some time and pain by telling you that you could get the same taste in your mouth by making out with a waitress at the Waffle House in Baton Rouge, minus the kidney damage from the cleanse diet.

These sorts of diets *are* tempting, but they DO NOT WORK. And the ones that make the most drastic claims about how quickly they can take off the pounds are the least effective *and* the most dangerous! Simply put, there is no secret formula, no magic combination of foods or ways to eat according to your blood or body type that will safely and efficiently take weight off. By following any diet that eliminates a food group from your eating plan, you are bound to be missing some nutrient.

For example, if the diet is lacking protein in the form of lean meats, chicken, fish, or eggs, then you will be missing the building blocks for most of the functions in your body. Yes, there are some proteins in beans and nuts, but not in the quantities your body needs, nor are they generally "complete" proteins. Eating incomplete proteins and ignoring complete proteins would be like buying shorts that are too small *and* don't have a zipper or buttons.

Another way to look at this is by skipping protein, you are building your body using wood but without nails to hold the wood together. Want a good image to put with this? If you've ever bought a boneless chicken breast and jokingly pictured it coming from a farm full of boneless chickens bobbing around in the middle of a field, that is what your insides are experiencing without enough protein.

I know, I know, seeing the latest diet crazes in such credible and inviting sources as the tabloids found at supermarket checkouts makes them pretty hard to pass up. It must be the headlines that suck us in: *"Woman probed by aliens sheds 3 dress sizes. Says weight loss is out of this world!"* Perfect! Let's all run out and get someone in an E.T. mask to give us a colonoscopy! Or how about: *"Farmer falls off tractor; is trapped inside cow. Claims living on dairy until rescued gets him in shape in just 5 days!"* So have we truly lost our minds? Apparently, the answer is, yes, we have.

Tim Wilkins

So, just what are some of the brilliant methods we think we can use to shed overnight what took us a lifetime to put on? Among them are names that I can't believe ever roped anyone into to trying them, like: the Caveman Diet, the Baby Food Diet, and the Tapeworm Diet. I'm not kidding; people actually have beef tapeworms put into their bodies. (More on that in a minute.)

Recently, there have been news stories about the Feeding Tube Diet. This is no lie. Some people, mostly brides-to-be, are having feeding tubes inserted by doctors. Next, they are fed a solution of fats, proteins, and water to sustain them while their bodies eat themselves. Wouldn't it be easier to get your dress a size larger than to be put into a medically induced walking coma? What's next, the Hospice Diet?

My favorite quote about the Feeding Tube Diet comes from Dr. David Katz, MD, MPH, of Yale University's Prevention Research Center, who said, "You could probably get the same effects as the Feeding Tube Diet by going on a 10-day cocaine binge. At least with the coke it would be more fun than the nasogastric tube." Don't give people any ideas, Doc, or the Tony Montana Diet could be next.

Some diets have names that really *do* make you want to try them, because they sound delicious, like the Twinkie, Hot Dog, and Lemonade Diets. Others, such as the Grapefruit and Watermelon diets sound like you could at least make it through them. And who could forget the Cabbage Soup Diet? This one is the worst of the bunch. That's because, while you might not lose weight on cabbage soup, you could lose friends! If the smell of cooking this green sewage doesn't keep people out of your house, then the stench flowing out of you certainly will.

On the other hand, if the 150 lbs. you are trying to lose is your good-for-nothing spouse, then get out the stock pot and start boiling. And while you're on this diet, stay away from campfires or you might take burning fat to a whole new level!

One of my favorites is the carbohydrate addict's diet. I agree with the premise of this one, because carbohydrates are drugs that some of us are hooked on, but "addicts," seriously? Isn't that a bit extreme? It makes us sound like we're junkies living on the streets begging for carbs to feed our habits. Someone comes out of the theater and we're slumped over on the sidewalk holding signs that say, "Will work for pasta" and "Can you spare a loaf of bread? Maybe just a slice, white, wheat…" Finally, you start stripping to pay for your spuds, using a stage name like, "I-da-ho." (C'mon, what would this bit have been without a bad potato pun?)

Then there's the South Beach Diet, one of my other favorites, and it actually works. You drive down to the beaches of Miami once a month and stare at people who should *never* be wearing thong bikinis! Trust me, you'll lose your lunch on the spot, and your appetite for days after. Anytime you're feeling even a little bit bloated, head down to Collins and 9th, just outside of Mango's, you'll find a hot dog vendor named Tito wearing a neon yellow banana hammock. One glance at him and is like putting a finger down your throat.

Actually, the South Beach Diet is not a bad way to go, but the name worked well for the comedy. The diet was originally created by Dr. Arthur Agatston, a cardiologist who wanted to reduce the cholesterol and insulin levels of his patients. It's basically an eating plan that includes all of the food groups, lean proteins, fruits, veggies, and whole grains. How they came up with the name South Beach Diet, I have no idea, but it was a better marketing plan than the Eat Healthy Diet. Who would possibly fall for *that*?

I want to spend a decent amount of time on this next gimmick, because not only has it been around a while and is still wildly popular, but also a lot of people I know have fallen for it. I'm talking about the Atkins Diet. Those I know who have gone on it have failed miserably.

Let me first say as proof of how unhealthy this diet is: Dr. Atkins is dead! Okay, so he died from a slip and fall on ice, but who's to say there wasn't a little bacon grease on the sole of his shoe from following his horrible diet plan? It is the original low-carb, high-protein, high-fat diet which has been reinvented over the years with little twists and new names to sell books.

You cannot convince me of anything about this diet other than what I have seen over and over: it will take weight off of you in a very unhealthy way, and put your original weight back on, plus a bit more, even faster than you took it off. On another note, the number-one killer of people in America is heart disease, and this diet is NOT recommended by the American Heart Association. Still not convinced? Oh, waitress, could we have the reality check please?

The Diet You cut your carbs down to 20 grams per day by not eating bread, pasta, rice, potatoes, etc. The rest of your caloric needs, at least from what I've seen with my friends, are ingested by removing the buns from double-bacon cheeseburgers and choking down two or three of those. Do this while wearing a big, dumb grin on your face and saying, "Dr. Atkins says I can have all of the protein and fat I want."

The Reality You start to lose pounds almost instantly in the first 7-10 days, during what is called the "induction phase." This is due to the drop in your insulin levels (blood sugar) from the lack of carbohydrates and the decrease in overall calorie intake that occurs when you remove the huge servings of bread, rice, and pasta from your life. You might experience some nausea, headache, sleeplessness, and bitchiness, while your cholesterol levels are going through the roof, but your pants are looser already!

The Diet According to the diet, in the second "phase," you can start introducing some quality carbohydrates in the form of high-fiber grains and veggies. What constitutes a high-fiber grain or veggie is right there on the list, but you've never really liked the taste of those so you kind of skip that part. Besides, the 5-15 pounds you dropped in the first two weeks has now slowed to maybe one or two pounds per week. So most people I know say, "Screw phase 2. Let's stay with what worked by living in the induction phase."

The Reality By cutting your carbohydrate intake to the levels suggested on the diet, you send your body into a state called "ketosis," in which it burns fat for energy. Sounds good, but not so fast… Your body normally uses those carbs to fuel your brain, heart, kidneys, and other vital organs. While these magical ketones are running through your body burning fat like those idiots who set fire to their cities after 12 guys they don't even know win a basketball game, they are also gaining toxicity by the day. So say hello to potential kidney stones, gout, and maybe even kidney failure. Hmm, what does a kidney weigh?

Then, of course, the cravings return and you eventually go back to your normal way of eating. This, from what I've seen over and over, happens quickly. There is no "maintenance" phase or gradual re-introduction of carbohydrates into the diet.

As I mentioned, if you knew how to eat high-fiber grains and veggies, you wouldn't be in this mess in the first place. It's belly up to the buffet and go time, bay-bee! The result is the famous yo-yo effect that comes from the insulin and hormone spikes associated with going off a diet. You practically killed yourself for months, and now your body goes into "pack-it-on" mode. I actually use a similar diet to help people put weight *on* before a sporting event. It's a modification of the ABCDE diet (Anabolic Burst Cycling of Diet and Exercise).

Simply put, if your eating plan doesn't have enough carbohydrates, then you are driving a car without gas. Eventually, that car will break down. Let's stay with that analogy, for the sake of learning something important, which is not all "car"bohydrates are the same. Processed flours, white rice, pasta, French fries, and sugars, are similar to that cheap gas you get from the Kwik-E Mart, where they mostly sell lottery tickets and cigarettes.

 What you want is the premium grade, expensive gas from the station with the shiny pumps and clean bathrooms. Those are the carbs with the high-fiber content. Multi-grain breads, pastas, and brown rice and a number of fruits and veggies all fall into this delicious and seriously good-for-you fuel category. Just remember:

- All of the fruits and vegetables that some diets tell you to avoid have a purpose; so eat them, in moderation. Too much of a good thing can become a not-good thing.

- Fats are not created equal, either. They are like witches in "*The Wizard of Oz*"; there are good fats and bad fats, so eat them in moderation. Nuts, salmon, avocado, olive, and grape seed oils…these and others are healthy fats that can change your diet and add big flavor.

- When it comes to carbs, it's important to know there are three kinds, one of which you should definitely avoid; they are simple, complex, and simplex. The one to avoid is simplex, which is what you get from kissing that not-so-sweet potato: I-da-ho, I-da-ho!

Without going into huge amounts of detail, I want to say that it's also important to know fiber is about more than just poop. It keeps almost every system in your body running smoothly, and especially, processing food to help you lose weight. So do your research and find ways to put a lot more fiber into your diet!

Other forms of this are the Low Carb Diet and the Meat and Bacon Diet, along with the latest twist, the Paleo or Caveman Diet. They all revolve around cutting your intake of carbohydrates in the form of bread, rice, etc., to nearly nothing and shoveling in a lot of meat. The Caveman Diet in particular focuses on dinosaur meat and getting most of your fiber from eating fossils. I could go on and on about how stupid this is, but can sum it up in two ways: 1.) Very few of the people on "*The Flintstones*" had good bodies, and 2.) Wasn't the life expectancy of the average caveman about 20 years? It's been over 20,000 years since the Stone Age, so before you fall for this crap, use a cell phone and order some common sense.

Again, I am kidding a bit about the Paleo Diet. It sounds silly, but some of it actually makes pretty good sense. Paleo rules say that if it comes from nature you can have it, sort of. Within reason, you can have all of the meat, veggies, fruits, and nuts you want. But what about grains, rice, potatoes, beans, and dairy? They come from nature, too, right?

The cave doctors and followers say you can only have food that can be eaten raw, except meat, pork and chicken. Of course, you can have also have milk raw, but they say that's a no-no. Yes, it's confusing. So read up on the diet to see what works for you and incorporate as many healthy foods as you can imagine that Barney Rubble might eat.

Meanwhile, back at the craziest diet of them all. When I was a kid, my mom used to say, "You eat like you have a tapeworm!" That meant I could eat and eat and never gain a pound. Apparently, someone else who heard that as a kid grew up to be either an overweight doctor or an underweight opportunist and got the bright idea: What if I *did* have a tapeworm and *could* eat whatever I wanted? Wouldn't that would be awesome? If it works, I could even charge people for the parasite and get rich! So he did. Ewww! People tried it, and it worked. The worm works its way down into your system, attaching as it goes and eating everything along the way. Then, and here's the magic, it continues to eat what you eat, so you lose weight. Perfect, right? Not so fast.

Eating for two is only effective when it's you and your future baby, because the baby knows how to share. The parasite (the tapeworm, not the baby) is truly eating what you eat, including all those important vitamins and other nutrients that come in your food, which could result in a dangerous deficiency for you. In addition to making you malnourished, your new alien friend can cause you to have cysts in your liver, eyes, brain, and spinal cord, and even kill you. The upside is there may be a period before you die during which you look great! (Back to the Hospice and Feeding Tube diets.)

There is a lot more throughout this book on how *to* get in shape, and we'll spend a lot more time laughing about how *not* to do it, but the important lesson is that there is no quick or easy way. You just have to do it! Before you dive into an overnight fix for a lifetime problem, stop and think about how far away the diet you are considering is from what you know to be the reality of healthy eating. Oh, and the only "Hollywood Cleanse" that should occur is flushing out all of the talentless reality "stars" and putting some *real* entertainment back on TV!

Stop being a guinea pig

When it comes to gaining muscle or losing fat, waking up or going to sleep, softer stools or stiffer stiffies, we'll take just about anything we think will get the job done. No need to do clinical trials or even double-check the math on the formula, just put out a claim about amazing results, stick it on a shelf, and we'll ingest it until the day it's taken off the market. We don't care what the side effects might be, as long as it does what it's supposed to do.

The best example of how we take things, regardless of their possible consequences, is illustrated by that list of disclaimers you hear at the end of most medicine commercials… "May cause sleeplessness, agitation, uncontrolled bleeding, kidney failure, increased heart rate, anxiety, and suicidal thoughts." And *that's* for a product intended to stop a runny nose! Good to know that when my insomnia has me in a clock tower with a high-powered rifle, at least my nose won't be dripping on the gun-sights.

At least most of the products manufactured for medical uses are tested for years and strictly monitored by the Food and Drug Administration (FDA) in the USA and the Health Protection Branch (HPB) in Canada. However, most diet aids and fitness supplements are *not* put under quite the same scrutiny until it's too late. Instead, they are watched about as closely as those shoeless brats running rampant in Wal-Mart while their halter- top-clad moms are busy trying to find a new baby daddy. This is because supplements fall under a law that exempts them from meeting the same "safety" standards as other drugs.

And the injuries we incur from taking them amount to hanging ourselves with that loophole.

To really drive this point home, since the supplement law was passed in 1994, over 51,000 new ingredients have been brought to market and only 170 have documented safety results. I'll save you the math: that's .3%, an even lower percentage than the number of talented musicians on a modern music awards show. Crazy to think about hitting an age where we can look back and say things like, "Back in my day, at least the bands used instruments, like synthesizers!" and "Take your meds, Grandpa, and please don't tell me about Depeche Mode again."

Even reading this cautionary info, it's still so tempting to take the latest wonder supplement isn't it? I mean, who can resist those amazing transformation pictures and overnight weight-loss claims? "Jeff lost 30 lbs. in just a few days…Stacy lost 24 lbs. in two weeks!" And *look* at those "before and after" pictures…yeah, before and after heroin, maybe.

Some of the pictures go beyond unbelievable makeover shots and instead look more like a 12-week snapshot of the evolutionary chart. For example, picture number one shows a man slumped over, sporting a huge belly, covered in body hair, and holding a club.

By the time you get to picture number five, he is in perfect shape, completely upright, and standing next to a picture-perfect woman in a bikini.

But, like they say, let he or she who is without sin cast the first kidney stone. That is to say, I've done my share of experimenting. I actually started my "supplementing" before protein powders were popular. Flashing back, I was a skinny kid, basically human wind chimes, and to remedy that I began making what I called "power shakes." After one too many times watching "Rocky," I started to make concoctions that were a delicious blend of milk, ice cream, peanut butter, and raw eggs. They were quite tasty, but this was also before I knew I was lactose intolerant or that the salmonella from the eggs could have killed me. Looking back, I wonder if it was my lagging physique that was keeping the ladies away or the noxious green cloud around me?.

Along the way, a buddy from the gym turned me on to amino acid pills. They were about the size of a baby's fist and who knows what they were really made of, but I was taking as many as I could. After all, if a little is good for you, a lot must be great!

I even tried a supplement the guy at the protein store suggested to get rid of the fat I gained from the last round of miracle shakes I was drinking.

It wasn't cheap either, so in my transformation I managed to gain three pounds of muscle, but lost 5% of my income. And, sadly, my "before and after" picture still had my ex in it. Evolution would come later… where did I put that cabbage soup?

Years later, while attending fitness expos, I would play trick-or-treat at all the booths, gathering up big bags of the latest untested potions and powders. I took them with the same level of scrutiny that a kid shows towards his Halloween candy loot. "Horny Goat Weed; Take this for more energy in your workout and increased blood flow to your downstairs," the package said. "Great!" I thought. "Better exercise and somewhere to rest my weights between sets!"

It's even easier to fall for supplements if they're labeled *herbal* or *natural*. Heaven forbid they were found in some remote village in the Amazon. "These remarkable tribesmen have no history of cancer after living for generations on the Acai berry!" Yes, but they also don't smoke or microwave their food. And carrying around a spear is far less deadly than clamping a cell phone to their ear. Put your wallet away; it's just another berry.

Things like Xango, Acai, and resveratrol, are also favorites of the multi-level marketing hucksters who tout these super-fruits as being everything from fat-burning to anti-aging, anti-cancer, and even an anti-virus for your PC. FYI, having a "doctor" backing these claims is meaningless compared to the results from perfectly good clinical trials.

If you want the benefits of a super-fruit, you're going to have to wait for Ricky Martin to be bitten by a radioactive spider. At least then you stand a chance of crime-fighting *and* a great soundtrack.

The ones we fall for the hardest are anything claiming to help us burn fat and lose weight. Guarana is one that shows up in most energy drinks and supplements. It both sounds impressive and gives you an extra bounce in your step. But that should not be a surprise; after all, it *is* herbal caffeine.

Appetite suppressants, such as fat- and carb-blockers, are among some my favorite so-called "miracle" supplements. Anything with the word "blocker" in the title conjures up a hilarious image to me. I imagine conversations among the cells in the body like, "Dude, I was in the lower intestine last night. I took a bunch of stomach acid and I was just about to digest this sweet bit of food, when a carb-blocker came and screwed things up."

The best example of a fat-burner gone bad in the last decade is good ol' Fen-Phen.

Originally when it was just "Fen," people could lose 10-15 lbs. by taking it while sticking to a decent eating plan. But when it was combined with "Phen" back in the '90s, the weight started falling off big time. What we learned later, however, was that some of the speedy weight loss was lung tissue and a heart valve or two. Between the kidney loss from the fad diets and this revelation, it's just a pound here and a pound there. But I guess that it somehow all adds up.

The warning you should take away from this information is that even after clinical trials and FDA approval, taking the easy way out in the form of "miracle pills" really *is* a way to stabilize your weight. Unfortunately, however, it may be the weight listed on your death certificate at the time of your autopsy. Not funny.

You can try anything that you think might help. But when you get right down to it, there is no substitute for time, a healthy lifestyle, and a little hard work.

Chapter 4

You Are What You Drink, Too

We have a major Coke problem in this country. We also have a major juice problem. Before you duck over to Urban Dictionary to see if I'm talking about cocaine and steroids, I'm not; although when it comes to our beverages, we could still use a healthy dose of rehab and a stern lecture from Dr. Drew.

 In addition to those "drinking" problems, we also have a major caffeine jones that adds literally a buttload (a clinical measurement for any quantity that causes our asses to grow) of calories to our diet in the form of fatty coffee drinks, too. All of this seems to slip our minds when we think about our daily calorie intake and where we can cut nutritional corners.

In Chapter 1, I mentioned keeping a food diary and the importance of making a list of everything you ate *and* drank. As easy as it is to forget the corner you shredded off of that donut in the break room to make it look like someone took a bite out of it, rendering it inedible to everyone else, it's even easier to forget about all the calories you drank, too. But these calories can seriously add up. Let's start with the juice, sodas, and energy drinks.

Totally juiced

It's time to talk about the crazy amount of so-called "fruit" juice we consume in America. I say "so-called," because the vast majority of the juice we drink has the audacity to proudly say on the label, "Made with 10% real fruit juice!" Ooh, 10%! Why are we so forgiving? Where else in our lives would we allow this?

You, dining out: "Hey, the waiter is coming with our dinner."

Waiter: "Please enjoy your meal. Tonight, the chef is serving steaks featuring 10% real meat."

If your boss paid you with 10% real money or the Chevron station switched to 10% real gas, you couldn't pay your bills or power your car; yet this practice seems to be okay with our beverages.

Of course, if the current plastic surgery trend continues, then the next generation will have 10% real parts, and we seem to be okay with that.

The most important fact about the remaining 10% of goodness in bottled juice is that it's missing the fiber and most of the natural vitamins that make it worth drinking, leaving less substance than a political speech. So with no fiber or vitamins and only a slight amount of fruit, what is the other 70-90% of liquid in that giant bottle we are paying up to $5 for? Why, it's the two cheapest things they could find to fill the container: water and sugar. And these empty calories are putting a lot more than 10% real flab on our bodies every year.

I used to laugh as a kid when the announcer in the commercials for sugary cereals would say, "Trix is part of this nutritious breakfast!" Meanwhile, the bowl of multi-colored sugar puffs would be next to a plate of eggs, whole wheat toast, juice, and a multi-vitamin. It was a part all right, the *unnecessary* part. Now, juice has become another way to add more empty calories to our already poor nutritional start to the day.

This is a HUGE area in which we can make a small change for big results in our kid's diets too. Capri-Sun is to juice what tanning beds are to the actual sun, artificial and just as bad for you.

And Sunny gives no Delight feeding it to me or my kids. Calling it Sunny D to make it more hip for the J-Lo generation is cute, but about as helpful as calling Charles Manson the C-man.

I have a strong feeling that one of the reasons this country's childhood obesity rate is higher than the kids at the skate park is because we throw them over-priced shot glasses of juice out of convenience adding hundreds of empty calories to their daily diets.

If we are giving kids juice pouches just to shut them up, Benadryl or duct tape works much better. (You know I'm kidding here; duct taping your kids is NOT legal in most states.) Tell them to go drink out of the hose like our parents told us.

Young or old, if we're thirsty, we need to find something to drink other than high-fructose corn syrup and Red Dye Number 5. If you drink "juice" because you want vitamins, then eat a piece of fruit or drink a glass of water and take a multi-vitamin.

Whatever you do, start reading labels and stop drinking this glorified sugar water. If you see on the label that fruit is not the major ingredient, then it's not fruit juice. A witch doctor waving an orange over a glass of water doesn't make it fruit juice.

Beat your Coke problem

In generations past, America has been known around the world for Levi's, baseball, apple pie, and Coca-Cola. Lately, however, those trends have taken an ugly turn as baseball is now known for steroids, and apple pie and Coca-Cola have contributed to the fact that fewer of us can fit in our Levi's without a strong friend to help us pull and tug.

While it's not fair to assign much blame to our once-in-a-while slice of American pie, it is fair to attach a few pounds of guilt to our national intake of soda. Our daily consumption of the dark and bubbly works out to almost 50 gallons per person per year. To give you an idea of how much that is, the average kiddie pool holds about 22 gallons. So picture Junior splashing in his floaties while you suck out all the liquid in the pool, refill it and suck it out again.

This stat is according to a survey cited in a 2010 *New York Times* article and, given that we are no slackers when it comes to overindulging, I have a feeling the survey was being gentle.

As with most statistics, that is an average; so take a minute to think here. If you are not much of a soda drinker, someone else is upping the average for you.

If you are, however, you might be drinking even more pop than an oil barrel full. With all of the extra sugar in those beverages alone, you run a higher risk of contracting Type 2 diabetes and gaining enough extra weight to make the next physician you have to see someone other than Dr. Pepper.

Let's break it down a bit shall we? One can of soda may be a mere 150 calories (all of which is sugar), but here's where it gets nasty. At my peak, I used to drink two to four sodas a day. While I'm no Rain Man, I know the average is three. Now, let's make the Algebra I teacher I had for three years proud and do a little word problem. Timmy has three cokes a day, five days a week, for one year, at 150 calories per serving. That's 3 x 150 x 5 x 52, which totals 117,000 calories from soda alone. Even if you can't do the math, you can rest assured that Timmy is steadily gaining one pound every week and a half.

If you're anything like I am, then you would much rather have eaten those calories. In fact, I would gladly trade those 600 empty soda calories I consumed once every four days for a trip to Chipotle to eat one of those burritos the size of a fat baby's leg. Mmm…fat, baby-leg burritos.

As if my nostalgic '80s references don't give away my approximate age or the era in which this book was written, allow me to cement things in stone. While this very chapter was being typed, the Big Apple went Big Brother by banishing Big Gulps, Super Big Gulps and Double Gulps. That's right, in late May of 2012, NYC pinched the straws of any sugary beverage larger than 20 oz., and cut people off like a cranky bartender.

And for those of you in states that still allow mega-drinks, I don't see the fight for keeping your rights to drink them as being the catalyst for the next Civil War. Of course, the South may "rise again," but after too many 44 oz. sodas or sweet teas, it won't rise very fast. Depending on how much ice is filling space in the cup, the average Double Gulp has over 650 calories. That's 163g (over 40 teaspoons) of sugar. Simply put, there is no good reason to drink that much sugar in one sitting. Not to mention that it's the reason so many people are missing teeth and why overalls sell so well in the South.

Does considering all of this make you want to make an easy change to your "lifestyle" that could pull pounds off right away? Then go back and read your diet diary. If you see that drinking soda is one of your downfalls, switch to drinking more water and watch the weight fall off. Before you know it, you could go from denim 1002s back to 501s in no time.

A load of (Red) Bull

Just a quick note about the other craze that has swept over us for the last decade: energy drinks. In an effort to not miss a single moment of our oh-so-important lives, we have been served a variety of multi-colored liquids intended to jack us up like Cougars waiting for the pool boy. One the most popular and best- marketed one has been Red Bull, the drink named after the Native American chief known for his life-long battle with insomnia.

Most energy drinks are nothing more than liquid crack; a lovely blend of sugar, caffeine, B-vitamins, and herbal speed meant to prolong the amount of time your eyes are open and your brain is popping. In addition to revving up your heart, lungs, and overall body function, the extra calories will have you haunted by another kind of "monster," Count Flabula.

For extra energy that lasts a lot longer, try sleeping and proper hydration, and cut down on the heavy carbohydrate and fat meals. If you absolutely *must* stay awake for a long drive or a bit more life, almost every energy drink on the market has a low-carb or low-calorie version.

Is it coffee or dessert?

Ever heard the old saying, "A sucker is born every minute"? The modern version of that should include: "At fancy coffee places across the world, suckers will pay up to seven dollars for a cup of hot, wet beans, cream, and flavored syrup." As offensive as it is to break down the cost of making coffee compared to what we pay for it, by the time your barista adds fat and sugar to the blend, the addictive nature of beast amplifies.

And there's no denying we *are* addicted. I've seen people dancing in line at Starbuck's while waiting for the fix, smacking their arms like Keith Richards getting ready to donate blood. Not to mention that we are gladly shelling out the same amount of money we could use on a healthy meal in the process. Even more disturbing is that we may not realize how our daily hookup to the Colombian IV is packing on the pounds.

I'm not picking on Starbucks; it's one of my favorite places. To be fair, we should include Seattle's Best, Caribou, Cosi, and even McDonald's, which has joined the mix because nothing says "trendy" like adding a "Mc" to the front of a food name.

It's not our plain coffee that is putting the pounds on us, though. According to recent studies, coffee by itself is actually a bit healthy for you, as it can ward off some forms of cancers and also Alzheimer's. (I think that's what it said; I can't seem to remember...) But what seems to be the diet downfall for many when it comes to coffee is throwing in a scoop of ice cream, drizzling on some caramel or chocolate syrup, and putting

whipped cream and crumbled Oreos on top.
Behold the Cookie-chino!

According to research done on the coffee habits of
New Yorkers, two-thirds of java drinkers went for
blended drinks that averaged about 240 calories.
Doing the math, that's about two pounds of
weight gain per month. When it comes to being
out of shape, does it really matter if you call your
extra belly roll either a "beer gut" or a "mobile
espresso machine"?

To make matters worse, it's hard to make good
nutritional decisions in a coffee house when have
to spend so much energy trying to order correctly
so you won't look like a dork. You're trying to
watch your waistline and you have a 20-
something tattooed hipster looking down her
pierced nose at you because you seem to have
forgotten the Italian word for "medium."

Not to worry, though, the coffee industry has
made it much easier for you to make good
choices.

All you have to do is use the word "skinny" when you order. How awesome is that? Whether you're ordering a Frappuccino, a Cappuccino, or an Al Pacino, just by saying "skinny," you can cut out more than half the calories. You get the same great flavor, but with nonfat milk, sugar-free vanilla syrup, and no whip. This means it's not topped with a layer of fatty foam or drizzled with a not-so-subtle hint of buttery caramel. Finally, a diet word that makes sense! The only way this could be any easier to understand would be if you said, "I'd like a Venti Cinnamon Dolce Latte, without the fat ass, please."

Booze it or lose it

Somewhere between six-pack abs and a beer gut is a party gone wrong.

All too often, we forget about the effects that drinking alcohol can have on our diets. Alcohol is one of those things that just seems to "get away from" us. And most times when you're drinking it, fitness or fatness is the last thing on your mind. A night can start off with a quick beer after work, then friends show up and the shots start flowing. Before you know it, you're reliving a scene from "*Dude, Where's My Car?*" or, worse yet, "*Coyote Ugly.*" (Note: a Coyote Ugly scene happens when you wake up next to someone so nasty you would rather gnaw your arm off and sneak out than wake up the other person by trying to free your trapped limb.)

At no point in that story were any of us ever thinking, "I wonder how many calories there are in what I'm drinking?" Nor were we giving the slightest consideration to how the alcohol might be slowing our metabolism, causing us to hold on to the calories from dinner longer than we normally would. And we definitely weren't giving even a passing thought to that meal we are going to have at Denny's or Waffle House at 3am, so we can "soak up the booze." If Denny's wanted to be more accurate in naming their dishes, then calling them Guilt Slam or Bender Breakfast Special would probably work just fine.

If none of the preceding has ever happened to you, the line for sainthood is the empty one on the right. For the rest of us, hopefully it's just once in every great while that we "party like rock stars." We know that line might sound awesome when you're screaming it at the start of a festive binge; but most rock stars die sad, bloated, and splayed across a toilet. I suspect that is not the way most of us want to be remembered.

But it's time to put the crazed, calorie-laden chug-fest aside for a minute because, for most of us, the larger obstacle is our daily drinking. And before we waste time discussing the down and dirty on martinis, most people are beer and wine drinkers, so let's start again with a little light math.

Let's say that on the low end we probably take in two beers or two glasses of wine per night, maybe five days a week. Yes, I'm rounding down and leaving out the weekend, like you did during your last physical exam, when your doctor asked how much you drink. But stick with me for a minute, please. Remember, we are working with two drinks x 150 calories (beer and wine) five nights a week times x 52 weeks a year = 78,000 calories per year. This is probably easier to understand: If you ate only lean proteins, high-fiber carbs, fruits, and veggies seven days a week for a year, you would still gain over 22 lbs. if you had two alcoholic drinks a day. (When I saw that number on the calculator, I said the same thing you just did: "Shit!")

Keep in mind that these calorie counts were calculated by a non-drinker using dainty little wine glasses. Real wine drinkers know that the flavors of a fine Cabernet or Pinot Noir come to life in a wide-mouthed glass that looks like a fishbowl (and doubles the serving size and the calorie count, unfortunately). In fact, I prefer a wine glass that Flipper would be comfy in and which triples the calories in each "serving."

Of course for the sake of fitness over flavor, you could switch to what I call the "workout beer," Michelob Ultra. At only 70 calories per bottle, it gives you two of the benefits of beer drinking, bad breath and frequent urination, while doing away with the calories or buzz of an actual drink. And it's the perfect drink to take in your water bottle when you go to the gym.

Many others who love to drink enjoy the so-called "hard stuff" (rum, bourbon, vodka), which usually goes down easier with "mixers" such as Coke, soda, Sprite, and Red Bull. It's often the mixers that make the harder liquors the best of two bad worlds for your diet. It's like having your main man ask you to hang out for the big game, then saying you "get" to cook for everybody.

Basically, you are getting the calories from the alcohol *and* the calories from whatever you mix it with, topped off with the slow-down-your-metabolism effect from the booze. Sorry, Captain Morgan, but you've just been demoted to the rank of Seaman.

Then there are the frozen and fruity drinks that look and taste delicious, and also pack enough of punch to make the next few drinks flow even easier. Mudslides, Blue Hawaiians, and the dreaded Pina Colada can each total between 300-600 calories. And that's in the adorable little serving sizes someone used in the laboratory, not the Slurpees on steroids found at most tropical party places. The average size I've seen for those drunken slushies is 32 ounces, which brings them in at between 2,000 to 3,000 calories apiece, or roughly four to six Big Macs!

Ironically, the only place you might actually waste away *is* Margaritaville. That's because a Margarita is one of the lowest-calorie drinks. I tried switching to Margaritas for the sake of my diet, but found myself doing a "spin" class that didn't include a bike or a real cardio workout. What was spinning was the room, so I put a foot on the floor and went back to good old H2O.

The point of all this is that your drinking should be in moderation if you *really* want to get in and stay in good shape. And, no, you CANNOT make cuts to your food intake to make up for your drinking. If that even crosses your mind, I've got a photo album to show you in which most of our family pictures were taken on the "12 Steps."

Beyond the bad diet choices and unwanted sexual encounters, drinking excessively can lead to a variety of other poor lifestyle choices, like smoking. My favorite band of ne'er-do-wells is the "I only smoke when I drink' crowd.

This is great logic; you get so drunk you forget you don't normally smoke! Nothin' washes down cirrhosis like cancer...

Sorry if this chapter reminds you of when you were a teenager and the cops showed up at your door just as your party was getting started. But at this point, you should have noticed that things are beginning to add up.

For example, if you have a cookie-chino in the morning, a soda with lunch, and a couple of drinks at night, you could be taking in an additional 1,000 calories a day. If you cut one or two of these drinks from your daily intake, then every two weeks, you'll be taking off a pound.

So what *does* that leave for you to drink? Well, as I mentioned before, there's always water. Throw some lemons, limes, cucumbers, or mint leaves in and pretend you're at a swanky spa. It's a calorie-free way to feel full, because processing water burns energy, and the more you drink, the more trips you'll make to the bathroom. The latter

means more walking and more calories burned.
See how it all works out?

Chapter 5

Cut the Cheese

I don't even want to think about how such a practice got started, but at some point in history someone obviously had a wild idea about getting underneath a cow and, voila, milk! As if that image isn't weird enough, sometime before refrigerators were invented, someone else was desperate enough to eat milk that had spoiled, which in my mind is even harder to explain.

It could be that the first artisans with this new food source were monks, and due to their vow of silence, no one bothered to speak up about how funky the spoiled milk tasted. So they just kept letting it rot longer and daring each other to eat it.

Centuries later, an obsession with cheese still exists. The milk from any animal that can be squeezed hard enough to start the process is turned into slices, cubes, or globs, and enjoyed worldwide.

 It isn't such an unhealthy practice on the surface, especially in places like Europe, where they eat tiny bits of cheese with tasty meats and veggies, enjoying it in moderation with pinkies raised.

In America, however, where we do everything "bigger and better," we are constantly looking for a new way to jam more of this gelatinous nutrition bomb into every recipe.

Dairy Council people are not going to like this chapter. I might even run the risk of pissing off the entire state of Wisconsin, but that's not really a big fear. If I see someone approaching me in the airport with a plastic wedge of cheese for a hat and an angry look on their face, I know it won't take a very brisk pace to get away, so let's get to the heart of the matter.

We eat too damn much cheese in America! Since 1970, the amount of cheese consumed in the good ol' US of A has tripled to 30 pounds per person per year. That's right, each year you are eating the number-one artery-clogging substance in the American diet in an amount the size of a large toddler.

Cue the Fat Bastard voice: "Umm, delicious…a tasty cheddar bay-bee. Get in my belly!")

Of course, I've vowed not to waste too much of our time giving medical pros and cons in this book. After all, we've been getting advice on cancer, heart disease, and diabetes for the last 20 years and could not care less. So let's just concentrate on what we *do* care about; for women, that would be fitting into a bathing suit for beach season. But guys who truly believe they're Brad Pitt as long as they can see their pee-pees beyond their guts are a lot harder to get through to. So just read along, and we'll try to plant some seeds of knowledge.

I would like to start by pointing out that it's not the cheese itself that is the problem; rather, that it is a "gateway" food. Cheese is to your diet what Benadryl is to crystal meth; almost good for you by itself, but we certainly tend to make a lot of bad things with it. Rarely does someone say, "I sure would like to put some cheese on this grilled chicken breast," or "Wouldn't a touch of cheese be lovely on these fresh veggies?" It's usually more like, "Hey, this entire loaf of bread sure would be tasty with cheese on it"…and… "This giant vat of pasta and meat needs cheese between each layer!"

Take cheese pizza, for instance. It really isn't *that* bad for you, as long as you have a small slice or two. But who the heck eats a *small* slice? Most of us eat pizza like we're Neil Armstrong: "One small slice for mankind, one giant pie for my face!"

If you get a "slice" in New York, it's the size of a laptop. You practically need tech support to eat it.

Ah, but for some reason, no matter how much pizza we eat, the cheese never seems to be enough. To fix that, someone got the bright idea to ask for double cheese as their two toppings. It was still not enough cheese though; so what did we invent? The stuffed-crust pizza! Cheese on top of cheese with bread stuffed with cheese. Seriously, why bother with the crust at all?

"Hello, Domino's? Send over a giant cheese wheel. No, screw the breadsticks, just a box of cheese and some laxatives."

In some cases, like with The Pizza Hut Insider, cheese overload is taken to yet another level by putting a layer between the crusts of the entire pie. Genius! The DEA had better hope the pizza industry never decides to go into the drug-smuggling business!

And if it's not the quantity or quality of pizza that we are eating that's getting us, it's the frequency with which we eat it. I know people who have it for lunch, dinner, and a hearty hangover breakfast, a few days a week.

If at any point someone in your house yells, "Who's your Daddy?" and you see Papa John, it's time to ease off the pizza.

Burgers are another food with which we just can't seem to get our fill of cheese. Apparently, there wasn't enough saturated fat in just one patty of meat and cheese, so our burgers have turned into towers of calories taller than almost any other food.

Step aside, Double Bacon Cheeseburger, you sissy health food. Meet the Hardee's Monster Thickburger. This monster features two one-third-pound slabs of Angus beef, four strips of bacon, three slices of cheese, and a load of mayonnaise on a buttered sesame seed bun.

The combo meal comes with medium fries, a large coke, and a souvenir stent for your blocked arteries. Calorie count: 1,420 for the burger, 540 for the fries, and a mere 400 for the drink to wash it down. Pick up the paddles and say, "CLEAR!"

And that isn't the only land mine for your thighs at Hardees, as they claim eight burgers with over 1,000 calories. And before you think it's only fast food joints that can get you, many restaurants with tables and real silverware are just dangerous. Get ready to sing *"Goodbye, Ruby Tuesday"* (2,000-calorie Colossal Burger). And say "Adios,

Applebee's," not to mention that the Outbacker Cheeseburger at Outback's has over 1,600 calories. Crikey, mate!

That's enough to put you Down Under. Add some fries and the mandatory oilcan of Fosters to that meal, and you've got two days' worth of food in one sitting. Oh, and if instead of throwing another "shrimp on the barbie," you decide to throw on some Aussie Cheese fries, you'll get another 2,140 calories. If I ate that much in one sitting, that's where I would be found throwing up... out back. Seriously, aren't fries glorious enough without coating them in cheese?

Now we move on to something that I myself find delicious and at the same time disgusting. That would be nachos. Yep, fried tortilla strips coated in melted cheese, meat, beans, sour cream, and salsa... done right. If you go for the kind at the ballpark or skating rink, the chips are probably fried cardboard and the cheese comes out of a ladle and looks more like thickened paint. Either way, you are looking at a gut bomb that you will pay for on your waistline and in your arteries and your intestines, as the nachos move through you like paparazzi stomping over Lindsay Lohan's garden.

If you are someone who routinely gets the "good" kind of nachos, you can try to make excuses all you want. "Oh, I'm getting my protein from the ground beef and fiber from the beans," you say. "And the tomatoes in the salsa are a natural cancer fighter," you might mumble as you shove nacho number 17 into your mouth. Sorry to tell you this, but you can argue your case in front of the Supreme Court or Diana Ross and the Supremes, but your Nachos Supreme is a big, fat loser for your diet.

Unless you're going to make nachos at home with light cheese, lean meats, and healthy veggie topping choices, here's how your diet breaks down when you order out. The lowest offender is actually Taco Bell at 420 calories, with half of those coming from fat. Topping out are the On the Border Stacked Border Nachos, which sport a muy gigante 2,740 calories, with 166g of fat and 5,280 milligrams of sodium. (In this case, if the fat doesn't put weight on you, the salt will have you retaining fluids like a waterbed.)

So before you are sucked into ordering a tray of nachos for the table, remember, even if the calories are listed on the menu and it sounds okay, that amount is probably per serving; which is six to eight chips. You're laughing with me right now, aren't you? Who the hell eats six to eight chips? So the next time you're browsing the apps on the menu, remember that nachos are just that…Not yo's!

Traveling: The Road Less Eaten

You're on the road again and, whether it's for business or pleasure, you've left the comfort of your kitchen and are at the mercy of restaurants run by clowns. You want to stay disciplined on this trip, but there they are, the Golden Arches. After a hundred miles of hunger, the deliciously greasy aromas are sucking you in more strongly than a sign that says Shoe Sale or a restaurant featuring sports on TV *and* scantily clad waitresses.

And, although travel shouldn't mean you have to take a vacation from eating right and practicing good health, unfortunately that's not the case for many of us. We leave for our trips as passengers and come back as cargo. As a comedian and speaker, most years I travel over 50,000 miles by plane and drive at least another 30,000. And out of necessity, or devotion to my diet, I have mapped the ins and outs of travel nutrition.

Probably the two most important factors that will keep you in shape on the road are knowledge and preparation. If you know what to eat and what *not* to eat at the various sit-downs and drive-thrus, you can make better informed decisions when you get there. To help you make good choices when you're on the road, many places have their nutritional information posted.

But that info can be harder to find than a clean bathroom. So until you can track that knowledge down for yourself in-store or online, I've cut a few research corners for you with these tips:

- **Have it your way** "Hold the pickles, hold the lettuce, special orders don't upset us"...Good! Because we're gonna be here a while. Don't be afraid to order your food the way *you* want it. Your special order may give the waiter or waitress an aneurism or the chef may spit in your food, but saliva has no fat.

- **Adding value** Which do you value more, your wallet or your waistline? Adding fries, chips, or larger sizes of everything for a small up-charge is not benefiting anyone, especially not you. Avoid the extras and, when possible, get some fruit or a baked potato with your fast-food sandwich.

- **Fried equals died** As in, you have just put your diet to rest by indulging yourself on your trip. The "carry on" from fried food won't store in your overhead compartment; this will be going in your seat! So eat fresh to feel fresh on the road. Order your meat, chicken, or fish grilled, baked, or roasted with sauces on the side. If need be, give special cooking instructions such as: easy on the oil, oil instead of butter, or sauce on the side. And, be aware that some restaurants like to drench things in enough sauce to make the BP spill in the Gulf look like an overturned sippy cup.

- **Avoid salad mistakes** Remember that salads are a nutritional trap to begin with, but they are even more so, on the road. Many are served with a breaded and fried meat and iceberg lettuce that has the nutritional value of wet paper. Fast-food salads tend to be empty when it comes to healthy ingredients, and full of calories from fatty toppings and dressings. So be sure to ask for lighter versions of your favorite dressings, and get them on the side.

- **FYI** Taco Bell's Fresco salad and the grilled chicken salads at McD's, Carl's Jr., KFC, Wendy's, and Chick-fil-A, all have under 500 calories. They are also low in fat and high in protein.

Why did the chicken cross the road? Because it was being chased by people on a diet! Mealtime-on-the-go holds an endless supply of menu items perfect for keeping you on track. These dinners tend to range from the chicken sandwich to the chicken salad to the chicken dinner.

Try to find chicken sandwiches that are made from chicken breasts and not miscellaneous parts shaped like a breast. This is easy in most states, except California, where they have gotten so good at substituting that you can't always tell which are real and which are fake.

> 1.) If you should happen across a restaurant with an actual chicken meal that offers side dishes…be careful! They are called "side dishes" because they will end up on your sides. (That, and calling them "butt dishes" didn't sound good in the marketing meeting!)

Keep in mind that mashed potatoes, mac n' cheese, and even some veggies are swimming in butter. Steamed veggies, and, if needed, rice or a plain baked potato are the way to go.

2.) Don't use a condiment. Sounds dangerous, I know, but they don't call it the "Mayo" clinic for nothing. Going commando on your sandwich by avoiding that glob of "flavor" could help keep your pounds down and your arteries clear. If it's flavor you need, every restaurant that has chicken sandwiches serves nuggets, and where there are nuggets, there are sauces. BBQ, honey mustard, or Sweet and Spicy, there are all sorts of ways you can add some zip to your bird on a bun without loading it with fat. Straight hot sauce and mustard are the lowest-calorie options.

The main at-home and on-the-go the dietary villain of the last few decades has been the dreaded carbohydrate.

With all of the bread baskets, rice, and pasta dishes, it's easy to lose sight of how many calories we're eating. Loading meals with carbohydrates is a big way for restaurants make money. Most chefs think of carbs as a Kardashian; they're bigger and look expensive, but, the truth is they are actually cheap and easy.

Carbs really haven't exactly gotten a fair shake with their fries because, like with cheese, it's often not the carbs themselves that are the problem. As I said before, it can be what we add to our carbs and how they are prepared, especially in the fast-food world, that makes them evil.

Baked and sweet potatoes are a great source of vitamins, minerals and fiber, by themselves. The damage is done by the butter, cheese, bacon bits, and sour cream piled on top. (Word to avoid: LOADED) Instead, try adding ketchup or BBQ sauce to your baked potato for the taste of French fries without the frying.

Brown rice is a great carb source, if it's steamed and not fried. If you do order fried rice, you need to know that when it's put in oil, it becomes the quicker picker-upper and absorbs an unholy amount of fat and sodium.

Pasta is considered the Carbosaurus Rex of the starch world. It can attack in two ways. First, beware of the portion sizes; and, second, creamy sauces are a real no-no. (I'm alfredo to think of how much fat is in some of our favorite dishes!)

Being aware of your carbohydrate intake on the road can be a huge challenge. If all else fails, use your travel time to cycle back a bit. Skip the pasta and potatoes, and double up on your veggies. Speaking of vegetables, they can be tough to keep up with when you're traveling. Whenever possible, get them steamed and not stir-fried or in a casserole. Raw is always good, just be sure to avoid fatty dips like Ranch dressing. Instead, think "skinny" dips like hummus.

And don't forget what I mentioned about drinks. Travel makes it even easier to forget about the 600 calories in your cookie-chino or sodas, or to let the floating party slip by as you add a couple extra grown-up drinks to your days. Water is always a good choice; just remember when you sit down to eat that you should drink a big glass to pre-fill the tank. (But be mindful, if you're on a car trip with others, of the amount of "pit stops" you'll have to make, because nobody wants to be *that* person.)

When all else fails, many convenience stores are now selling fruits, nuts, vegetables, protein bars, and shakes. With snacks, be sure to keep a watchful eye on "boredom eating."

A lot of us have this burning desire to do something with our mouths at all times. And, while I'll leave the "why" up to Freud, I will tell you that just because you're not talking doesn't mean you need to be eating. If no one on either coast can take your call, try sugar-free gum instead of mindlessly stuffing your face.

When it comes to portions, there is no shame in sharing an appetizer and an entrée. More than 70% of entrees were recently found to greatly exceed portion standards. And not only is sharing a great way to stay in shape, but it will also save you money on gas by keeping you from weighing down the car. Cha-ching!

The most crucial thing to take off of your travel menu, however, is pressure. Traveling is a great time to enjoy the variety of flavors special to the area you are visiting. (But, remember, just because a state is famous for its pork sandwiches is no excuse to be a pig.) Enjoy the tastes of the road in moderation, so you can expand your culinary horizons without expanding your waistline. This will mean that you can bring back new clothes from your trip as souvenirs because you *wanted* to, not because you needed bigger sizes.

Do your best to eat right and take care of yourself but, more than anything else, use what little time you have traveling to relax. Try your best not to overeat, and be aware that you can return to your mostly full-time healthy eating habits when you get home. And, if you *do* find yourself super-sizing anything on the road, then be ready to have your road trip turn in to a *guilt* trip.

Chapter 6

Cheat in Moderation

I'll bet seeing that as a chapter title really grabbed your attention! No need for cardio workout today, your heart rate is already into its fat-burning zone. I have to admit my wife wasn't crazy about seeing the title of this chapter, either, and after glancing at my notes she wanted to know who the hell "Pam" is. Turns out that Pam was the name of the cooking spray written on the top of a shopping list.

For the record, I'm not hooking up with Pam or Mrs. Butterworth. And I'm also not talking about the cheating that has some toothless inbred charging the stage on Jerry Springer. I'm talking about the kind of cheating that we all do on our healthy lifestyles.

Some people do it because of a lack of willpower or discipline, and some do it out of necessity.

People in the know do it for another reason, however.

They do it because occasionally splurging with your favorite foods can be a great way not only to keep your sanity, but also to reset your body into fat-burning mode. The moment of honesty here is that there is only so much of what most people consider diet food that you can probably eat without mentally snapping and taking hostages until your cheesecake comes. I've seen that happen too often, and am aware that occasionally letting the steam off on the diet pressure cooker can keep you happy and marching calmly on your path to good health.

Part of the difficulty in sticking to the right things to eat is that, at times, it can seem so damn boring. Since very few of us have the skills to be the Food Network's "*Next Big Star*," what we end up with is "*BAM!*" chicken and broccoli followed by "*BAM!*" egg whites. That might sound tasty to someone who's been eating bugs and rice on Survivor Island, but after a few weeks of eating this kind of meal every day, I feel like my diet is a *bored* game called "Monotony."

The only recipe this behavior can be is one for disaster, because after a few days on any new eating plan, your body starts missing more than flavor and variety. It starts missing the rush that it's used to getting from the truckloads of carbohydrates (bread, pastas, cereals, etc.) normally found in most of our diets.

What you are doing when you suddenly change to a healthier way of eating is like rehab for your body. And, while cold turkey is a good lean protein, eating it exclusively can be a hard way to get in great shape. So, give yourself a little break. To do that, a purposeful pause for pasta or whatever forbidden delight you crave is a great way to shock your body into keeping the pounds coming off.

If you think about the times you've tried to diet, they usually went like this: You didn't need to cheat on the first few days of your new eating plan because, although you felt hungry, you really weren't suffering *that* much. Not to mention that in the first week or two, the weight was really falling off, so you thought you could stick it out.

But dieting can be like running through the house with an armful of clothes from the dryer. The pounds come off your body like that trail of socks and underpants you dropped between the dryer and the bedroom. Out of the gate, you might have shed anywhere between five and 15 pounds and you felt unstoppable.

The frustration kicked in, however, when things slowed down and you were still eating that dreadful *healthy* stuff. That's when the reality of "dieting" set in. Sadly, most, if not all, of what you lost was water weight, and when the actual fat loss started, the pounds coming off slowed to one to two per week. Or, even more sad, the weight loss might even have stopped all together. Bitch!

However, by having a "cheat meal" once every week or two, you can trick your body into thinking you've been rescued from Starvation Island, and it can go back to processing and using calories as usual. Then you return to eating healthy and losing weight. Yes, I really said that. No other bullshit diet will tell you that.

I will also repeat "every week or two," because treating yourself to dessert at the end of each day for being good is the same mistake that made a generation of kids pudgy: "Clean your plate and you can have a treat." Thanks, moms! Maybe you could have taught us how to use sponges and dish soap instead. That way, you would have your precious plates clean and we might not be fighting an epidemic of Type 2 diabetes.

The reality of living a healthy lifestyle is that a lot of the successes that we enjoy won't come from the "plates" we load on weight machines, but from what we load on our dinner plates. As I said before, it doesn't matter how hard you work out, if you are wrecking it with your food intake, then you are spinning your wheels at best and, more than likely, going backwards. Healthy eating is 80% of the battle in achieving a good weight.

I know it's going to be hard, but it's time to make a move. Call the Domino's guy and tell him it's over. Those late-night calls to come over for something hot have got to stop. Say you need your space but you can still be friends; and he can still come over once in a while, just not every night like he used to. Tell him you'll call when you're in the mood to cheat.

By taking the time to plan your meals, and your cheat meals, you set yourself up for success in every direction. This practice gives you something to look forward to, and you can *plan* the joy rather than letting it happen with reckless abandon. Just remember there is a big difference between veering slightly off track and derailing. It's *not* called "The Little Engine that Could Eat a Pizza by Itself."

So before you let your cravings turn you into a sweaty-headed Bobcat Goldthwait from "*Police Academy*" let a *cheat* meal, or cheat day, keep you from going to the crazy place. In other words, every once in a while, it's okay to stay on track by letting loose and enjoying some of the foods you love to eat.

I'm not suggesting that you binge like a vampire locked in a blood bank, but treating yourself within reason can be very effective. Cravings are normal. Around that time of the month, maybe it's chocolate you want. After a breakup, maybe it's a pint or ten of Hagen Daz while you lie under the covers watching "The Notebook." Guys know that hot wings and sports are joined by nature. The point of life is to live and to live, as healthily *and happily* as possible

Get into swapping

I figured I've already roped you in with sexual innuendo in this chapter, so why not stick with the theme? Maybe my next book will be a dirty novel about losing weight on protein shakes. I'll call it "*50 Shades of Whey.*"

As with the earlier cheating reference, however, the swapping I am talking about has nothing to do with multiple couples playing drunken games of Twister that eventually lead to neighborhood cookouts where no one makes eye contact. I'm talking about how small changes you make to foods you already love can cause a big difference in your calorie intake *without* compromising the flavor.

I have to admit that you might see some of these tips and say, "Could you possibly suck any more fun out of eating?"

Others among you might be thinking you could try them every once in a while. But however you look at them and whatever you try, they are options that over time could cut a hundred or so calories from your diet every day or every week, and lead to a big weight loss over time.

This first is one of my favorites. For years, my morning breakfast ritual has been exercising apartheid with my eggs; egg-gregation if you will. Call me backwards, but I have an "egg whites-only" policy with my meals. That's not totally true, because I actually use one yolk for every three whites, but by cutting out those two yolks, I'm dropping about 15g of fat, or 135 calories.

(Rain Man says, "Yeah, four days a week, 52 weeks; definitely cutting 28,020 calories per year.) This high-protein breakfast is a great way to start your day at home and an even better way to live on the road. And when it comes to recipes that call for eggs, you can use two egg whites for every whole egg.

This next swap takes the cake, literally. If a recipe calls for oil in a batter, as many cake recipes do, switch out the oil for applesauce. Switching one-half cup of vegetable or canola for applesauce will save over 900 calories, and keep people from poking your tummy like you're the Poppin' Fresh Doughboy.

Staying with the subject of cake and our theme of buzzwords that tell you that you are making a dietary mess-up, if you need dessert, go *Angel* Food cake over *Devil's F*ood cake. Easy enough to remember: eat Devil's food cake and your diet is going to hell. To make Angel Food cake even better, try fresh berries and fat-free whipped cream on top. (Quick recipe sidebar: Using a cold blender, a dash of vanilla, and evaporated milk, you can make your own whipped cream, fast, and it will be fresher and tastier than anything that comes out of a can.)

See, I just said it's okay to have cake. Yay, cake! As with anything else, though, watch your portions. Don't treat your cake like you're a baby on its first birthday, jamming pastry in every hole as fast as possible. Also, beware the giant piece of cake at the deli when you're out with friends. You know the one: It's maybe a one-inch wide sliver, but it's also eight inches high with a chocolate mousse Mohawk. Inevitably, the skinny friend who orders it to share with the table gets four spoons and takes only one bite, and you end up killing it with one other person. If that does happen, be sure to force-feed a few extra bites to little Miss I Just Wanted a Taste for good measure.

Another easy swap-out is exchanging low-fat yogurt for sour cream.

What's one glop of spoiled milk for another, right? As long as you get plain yogurt, you'll barely notice the difference, but your waistline will. Changing out one cup will shave off over 300 calories. So switch out your next dip mix with yogurt, add some veggies to dunk along with the chips, and there's another pound off.

This next one is a really big change and an easy place to cut back without much effort. Using ground turkey (specifically, ground turkey breast), instead of ground beef in recipes will cut the calories by half or more. One complaint is that turkey is less flavorful than ground beef and, for the most part, that's true. I have also heard that your taste buds become less sensitive to flavors after you're *dead*! Enough with the saturated fat already, add a little hot sauce or extra seasonings to the turkey. Your arteries will thank you, and maybe the hot sauce will speed up your metabolism while you sweat it out.

Cooking at home is by far the best way to become thinner while your wallet grows fat. It usually costs one-half or less to cook at home versus eating out, which equals more money for clothes you will need to buy when the weight falls off. Notice I said cooking at home and not home cooking, the latter which implies Nana's comfort food made with love and a snow shovel full of butter.

As I mentioned in the travel nutrition chapter, the only people being made "happy" with meals we eat out are restaurant owners and cardiologists. By cooking at home, you can monitor all of the ingredients and their calorie counts and qualities, so you know what you're getting in your food.

One thing that even the fanciest restaurants use in mass quantities is butter. From the finest French chefs to Paula Deen, who puts a little behind each ear to keep that yummy scent alive, butter is the ingredient that binds cooks together. When you're cooking at home, you can cut big calories by using non-stick spray, oil in a mister, and even low-salt broth to keep foods from sticking to the pan.

I've said it before but it bears repeating, we eat way too much pasta. Why? Because it's inexpensive to make and damn tasty. For a big slash at calories and a huge switch in flavor, use thin-sliced squash in place of noodles in pasta dishes and lasagnas. If you're not ready to step up to the primavera plate, ease your way to better health by using all or some whole wheat noodles.

They are more filling in smaller quantities, and the added fiber helps you burn more calories as the body works harder to digest it.

To cut some calories *and* add some zip to your mashed potatoes, try mixing in half of the amount of your cooked spuds with well-steamed cauliflower. This not only cuts the carbohydrates in your side dish, but sneaks in a bit of much-needed vegetables, too. Also, ease off the butter and heavy cream when mashing. Instead use 2% low-fat milk, almond milk, or a dollop of low-fat sour cream to make your taters fluffy.

There are hundreds of tiny tweaks you can make to your foods that will make a huge difference in your calorie count and overall health. So don't be afraid to blow the whistle on your favorite foods and call for a substitution.

'Tis the season…Surviving the holidays

Let's face it. If you look hard enough at the calendar, you can always find a holiday or some random excuse to stuff your face. There are the easy ones like Thanksgiving and Christmas, all that chocolate on Valentine's Day, and tacos on Cinco de Mayo.

There's corned beef, cabbage, and green beer on St. Patrick's Day and ham on Easter; we'd even consider Fried Groundhog if someone could make it a day off from work.

While you might be able to avoid falling completely off the wagon or allowing yourself a cheat day on some of the above, we seem to engage in a full-on feeding frenzy from late October to February. After all, we're wearing winter clothes for a few months, so who's gonna see the weight gain?

When the holidays descend upon us, it seems easier to forget our healthy eating and workout regimens than it is to find a parking spot at the mall. I know in my family the excuses start flowing at the first harvest of candy corn and don't let up until the boxes of Valentine's chocolates have nothing left in them but wrappers and half-eaten pieces with centers that unexpectedly went 'gush.'

I know you're thinking, "It's Christmas, Mr. Scrooge. Can't we have a bit more porridge?" I'm not here to ice your Christmas cookies with sprinkles of humbug but, managing food during the holidays is one of the ways I've kept myself Tiny Tim.

That said, let's look at a few tips for the season that will help you keep your holidays merry and *light*.

The first survival method would have to be (drum roll, please) moderation. Instead of plowing the

buffet table clean with your face, try sampling a
little bit of everything from the cornucopia. Limit
yourself to one or two servings, not helpings and
remember that lifting heavy plates of food does
not constitute a workout.

Avoid anything mashed. These are foods that
chefs use to get rid of all that extra butter and
heavy whipping cream which was about to go bad
in the fridge. It's also a time when people break
out their "family" recipes, sharing generations of
heart disease with their friends. A handy piece of
insight to ponder is that we don't have the family
"body shape" because of a genetic malfunction,
we have the same big butts and hips from having
the same family eating habits!

And, adding insult to injury, bailing out that gravy
boat like a deckhand on the Titanic doesn't do
your waistline any favors, either.

While we are on the subject of family recipes,
let's quickly touch on something usually found on
the table beside the potatoes: casseroles. Any dish
that has the word "ass" in it is not health food. So

pass on these foods whenever possible. Yes, that means the broccoli cheese and green bean casseroles, too.

Don't be fooled by flecks of green in the dish; it is *not* good for you. Think of that casserole as one of those forests in a scary movie; it might look like an inviting place to take a walk in the woods, but you know deep down that it's not going to end well.

Another source of hidden calories that we talked about is alcohol, happily referred to as "holiday cheer." Not only does the free-flowing liquid quickly add extra calories, but Yuletide mixers like eggnog are a double-whammy. I'll go on record as saying that I like the flavor, but I have a question: I know what an egg is, what the hell is a nog? This seasonal favorite doubles the fat, carbs, and, subsequently, the calories of the already potent shot of whatever you started with. And it slows down your metabolism, which doesn't help your body burn through the huge meal you just had.

If you must have a couple drinks, there are some delicious low-fat nogs out there. As for me, I'm still waiting for them to come up with an "egg-white" nog that is high in lean protein but still contains yummy rum.

The last piece of the holiday survival puzzle is maintaining your workout regimen. I know that with shopping, company parties, traveling to visit your in-laws, and the holiday change in gym hours, keeping up with exercising can be a real challenge.

But sneaking in an occasional workout or at the very least a few extra-brisk laps through the mall, will help to put another Yule log on that fat-burning fire. You might complain at first about how far away your parking spot is, but count those steps with pride.

Working out can also help you maintain your sanity. By the eighth day of Christmas, I might be wandering the streets wearing nothing more than a strategically placed Santa hat, if it weren't for an occasional trip to the gym.

Whether you decide to stay focused on your eating and exercise plan or throw caution to the wind by rolling everything in to one massive New Year's resolution, enjoy yourself. Either revel in your healthy dedication or let it go and EAT! Carrying a 40-pound sack of guilt with you on the treadmill won't make getting back to your workouts any easier.

Chapter 7

Sticking to It

I have to admit that I don't exactly bounce into the gym every day looking like Tigger after a six-pack of low-carb Red Bull. As with anyone else, I have my days when finding the motivation to work out and eat the right foods is a major task. Even the perfect-body people on the covers of fitness magazines have told me in strictest confidence that they have their moments of weakness, too.

Many people have come to me over the years for help in taking the first step towards or getting past a sticking point with their weight-loss goals.

So in an effort to help, I've tried to think about some of the things that have kept me trudging forward over time. And that's what it's really about, making an attempt to do the right thing for yourself, every day. Sure, you might fall back a little or take some time off, but continuing to work at it is the key.

There's an old joke in the cruise industry about how, on a seven-day vacation, people board the ship as passengers and leave as cargo.

That's because a cruise is a floating Bacchanalian orgy of food and drink. Think three meals a day, along with 24-hour pizza and sandwiches, topped off by a midnight buffet. It's no wonder the toilets on cruise ships need jet propulsion to get the job done! A cruise sounds like fun, but with a big-enough spoon and some determination, you can undo a year's worth of dieting in a few days.

You know as well as I do that falling off the wagon is one thing, but being dragged behind it is quite another. The longer you stay in a pattern of unhealthy eating, the harder it becomes to go back to on track. So if you do fall back a little or "hit the wall," here are some tips to keep moving.

Set goals

Plain and simple, setting a goal gives you something to shoot for. It can be the weight you want to lose, the pair of pants you want to get back in (yours or someone else's), a health goal like a lower cholesterol number, or a entering a competition like a race. Whatever the goal is, it needs to be realistic and, more than anything, specific. Also, as is the case with anything fitness-related, it has to be safe.

What I mean by specific about your goals, for example, is to say to yourself, "My goal to change my eating habits is to____."

It's not enough just to say, "I'd like to drop a few pounds," or "I'd like to *feel* better." Temporarily *feeling* better is what gets a lot of us *into* trouble. Pizza makes me *feel* better. A weekend hanging out on the beach drinking with friends makes me *feel* better. At least, it does temporarily. While we are enjoying and justifying life's little pleasures, all is right with the world. Unfortunately, however, every life has a Monday and whether your hangover is a headache or having your gut *hanging over* your belt, reality soon sets in.

You can even take your goal-setting a step further by going beyond a goal to an intention. An intention is an aim that guides your purpose. I'm certain your intention for losing weight goes deeper than, "I just want to see my toes again." Maybe you want more energy to play with your kids or you miss being more active. To get in touch with your intention, dig down to the root of what you *really* want, and you will have a much greater chance for success.

Give me a freakin' break

Better yet, give yourself a break. One of my favorite parts in any comedy movie is the boot camp scene in "*Stripes*," when John Candy's very overweight character explains that he joined the Army because his doctor said he swallows a lot aggression…and a lot of pizzas, too.

He figured the Army was a good place to get rid of his aggression and burn off a few pounds in the process.

The point is, for many of us, weight gain has an *emotional* component that is holding us back, as opposed to a lack of knowledge or dietary discipline. So when it comes to change our eating habits in order to look and live better, it helps to let some things go. You're going to slip up, but dieting is like learning to ice skate. If you fall down, get up, grab the rail, and laugh at yourself until you find your footing, then move forward until you can let go again. Obsessing over food mistakes or life's little indulgences is like having an ice skating friend who keeps grabbing at you every time he or she starts falling. Why should you get dragged down because Little Debbie was born without coordination? (Yes, I used Little Debbie for a reason.)

Time to be a total burnout

You've probably been thinking, "This book has managed to suck the fun out of eating. I wonder when it's going to finish the job of wrecking my life and start insisting that I exercise."

How could I possibly let you down? Go put on your yoga pants or sweats, as if you're not already wearing them, and let's talk about working out.

I know you already hate the term "working out." How could you not? It's got the word *work* right in it. I'll admit that exercise isn't easy and, for some people, it never becomes *fun*. It takes time, effort, and more consistency than most of us put into flossing or eating fiber.

I've visited entire regions of the country where the people don't exercise. On one trip to a small town in the South, I asked the hotel's front desk clerk, "Do you have a gym around here?" He answered without hesitation, "We do, but he's on vacation."

If you really don't like exercising, this may be encouraging: I strongly believe that it is not *the* most important part of burning fat and getting in shape. If I were to set a ratio of the importance of working out to lose weight and be healthy to eating right to lose weight and be healthy, it would probably be 20/80.

If you've ever looked over at a group of construction workers and seen a few who were quite overweight there's your answer. If eight hours of hard labor in the blazing sun won't keep you trim and fit, then there must be something more to this weight-loss thing.

So you can't just eat whatever you want and work it off doing a couple of laps around the building at lunch with the girls in the office.

Sorry, but walking at a leisurely pace and stewing in your own juices for the rest of the afternoon isn't going to work off the 40 grams of fat in the Caesar wrap you have waiting at your desk.

You can, however, enhance the process of slimming down and feeling great with exercise. So let's talk about *that* 20% of the fat-burning puzzle. Since regular exercise or even any exercise probably isn't a part of your current lifestyle, let's ease into it with everyday activities that set the bar extra low, so you can start feeling a sense of accomplishment. Rather than put all that pressure on yourself to do 100 sit-ups or crunches a day, make sitting up to turn off the alarm clock an accomplishment. Yay! You did it! Don't think of whacking the snooze button as laziness; think of it as another rep every nine minutes.

Take turns hiding the remote control for the TV from your significant other. You'll do pushups getting down on the floor to look under the couch, and your pulling muscles will get a workout when you dig under the cushions. Don't forget the cardio routine you'll practice when you get up to change the channels.

And might I suggest exercising while you watch Reality TV? After all, there are only a few seconds of those shows worth watching, so try to time them for the top of your sit-ups.

As an added bonus, most Reality TV shows will make you sick to your stomach, meaning that "The Real Housewives of Who Cares" suddenly becomes a great appetite suppressant!

For the ladies, I suggest using public toilets more often. This may sound like one of the most bizarre fitness tips you ever heard, but I am told that to keep from touching the seat, you actually do partially squat and hover a few inches above it. This is a phenomenal fitness move that works your legs, butt, and calves. Two of the main reasons you have better lower halves than men are wearing high heels and hovering.

This brings me to another great tip…Ever thought about "cross-training," guys? That's right, if wearing high heels is good for your calves, then put on a dress and some sensible heels and hit the treadmill.

The "push-away" is actually one of the greatest moves in married fitness. When your other half comes on to you with those nightly advances, turning him or her down is actually a workout. One night, push your other half away using your arms, and the next night, use your legs. Always keep your core tight.

Speaking of resistance exercise, I can't emphasize enough the importance of lifting weights or doing machines. Too many women are reluctant to try this, because they think they will develop "big muscles." Look around the gym, ladies. There are probably a ton of guys in there who lift every day and still can't manage to become buff. So you're not going to hit the weights a couple times and wake up looking like the Terminator. Women are not equipped with the testosterone to build muscle in great quantities. But the exercise you do to building muscle is what will help you burn fat.

That's right; muscle is the engine in your body that burns calories. That's why lean people tend to stay lean. Every pound of muscle you build will help burn an additional 30 to 50 calories per day. One of the biggest myths about losing weight is that you can do it only through cardiovascular work like walking, running, or biking, or that you can *sweat* it off. Cardio helps burn some of it off, but any weight lost with sweat is just water which is replaced as soon as you take a drink. Building muscle, however, can help you take weight off and keep it off.

Besides the fact that most people think exercising sucks, what are the most common excuses for not doing it?

- I don't have the time.

- I don't know what to do.

- I can't stay motivated.

Let's tackle these one by one, and see if we can't beat them down a bit.

I don't have the time

This one, I get, sort of. We all have busy lives. You get up in the morning and rush out the door to a full day of work, and come home at night buried in things to do before you get to sleep. But there has to be *some* free time in that mess. For example, is there any way you can sneak out early in the morning and hit the gym before the family wakes up? That may seem like a lot to ask on some days, but at other times, it will be like an hour at a Zen retreat. Nobody will be yelling your name or asking you for anything, so it's just time that's all about you! If you are a parent of little ones, you know that kind of quality "me" time hard to come by.

As I mentioned before, what about working out while you're watching TV? Whenever I ask people what their favorite shows are, they usually say they don't watch TV. But I don't exactly have to water board them to find out their 10 must-see shows. Guess what? They have TVs at the gym now.

Plus, you can actually work out in front of the TV at home. It's convenient, and no one will see or judge you, no matter *what* you're wearing. Think of it as being in the Fitness Protection Program.

The reality of a good workout is that it can be done in about 20 minutes, if you hit it hard. Are you telling me you can't find 20 minutes? Maybe you could stay off of Facebook for that amount of time a few nights a week and motivate yourself to hit the weights, instead.

I don't know what to do

You say you don't know what to do. For starters, there's this crazy new thing called the Internet. Maybe you've heard of it? If my kids can learn how to play a guitar and take apart the engine of a '72 Mustang by watching YouTube videos, then you can certainly find easy ways to get in shape. As a matter of fact, I put "workout routines" and "proper exercise form" into Google, and my search was hit on more than J-Lo at a Cinco de Mayo parade. It's there; you just have to look.

Another great method for learning your way around the gym is using a personal trainer. I usually see a bit more resistance from guys to this idea, because the gym is one more place we would rather wander around looking like idiots than leave our egos in the locker room and ask for help.

If you can't afford a trainer full time, you could just get one to set up a program and run you through it a few times. Actually, many gyms will have a trainer show you around the machines when you sign up. Jump on that! Learning the right way to do things will really help you to have good workouts or, at the very least, help you not to look like a piece of spandex having a seizure.

Another great reason for both men and women to get a trainer is that having someone to work with who is hot and in shape can be a big motivation to push yourself a little harder.

I can't stay motivated

If you really don't like working out, why suffer alone? Remember what they say, "Misery loves company."

Having a workout partner can serve some very important functions. The first of these is accountability. If knowing someone is waiting for you is the only way you'll actually go to the gym, then so be it. Motivation is another thing that a workout partner can add to your training arsenal. Finding the right partner or partners can be a real challenge, but it's really just a matter of figuring out what you want to achieve by working out with that person.

I have a number of training buddies who are like my wife's shoe collection, appropriate for every occasion. There's my "getting big" buddy, the one who yells and grunts a lot. Let's call him "the pump." I don't call him often. My body can't handle that level of workout for great lengths of time and, frankly, it's embarrassing. By day three of working out with him, my joints sound like a bowl of Rice Krispies.

Then there's my strict form and high-reps partner for when I feel like training without injury, but still want to get big results. Plus, I always seem to learn something from this guy in the form of a new move or the right way to be doing an old move. He's kind of my utility partner, like that pair of strapless flats the Mrs. likes to wear when we have to do a lot of walking. (I'm glad she's not one of those women who wears her "hooker heels" to an amusement park and says, "I can't walk in these." Where do women like that *think* they're going?)

Last, there is my cardio partner. Along with this person comes not only the intense motivation to do endless amounts of walking, running, and stepping, but he also has good conversation skills which the "grunter" and the "repper" just can't seem to muster.

Oddly, they are all good nutrition buddies, which is even more important. Going out to eat with them is effortless. Not only is it not embarrassing or difficult to stay on my eating plan, but if I wait until after they order all I have to say is, "I'll have the same." And I know I won't have someone sabotaging my hard work by talking bad about the healthy food I'm eating.

Finding the right workout partner can be harder than finding an exercise bike that doesn't chafe your crotch, so here a few simple guidelines that can make it an easier task:

- Find a partner with similar intensity, not necessarily similar strength, to yours, because it's a mental push that you are looking for.

- Find a partner with similar knowledge. This will keep the situation more buddy-buddy and less trainer-trainee.

- Find a partner with good hygiene. You are going to be in some pretty precarious positions as a spotter or spottee, so it's best to have some good-smelling parts. I know the last distraction I want to deal with when I'm on the bench press is a toxic-crotched workout buddy doing a squat over my face!

• Find someone reliable who will actually show up, and be on time!

Other great reasons to get a workout partner are safety and stability. Working out is like having a baby; it hurts. (By the way, if childbirth is so natural, why do women need to spend eight weeks in Lamaze class learning how to breathe?) Having someone there to remind you of what you should be doing can be a great safety tool. Of course, you are thinking, "I can just watch myself in the mirror." But we both know that mirror is used for checking yourself out only when you're not too busy checking out the people around you. So bring someone with you to watch your lifting form, and that will free you up for the important things.

In describing the perfect workout partner, I've also described the ideal mate, which in a sense is true. The best workout partners are long-term.

You can't be jumping from partner to partner without causing some problems. I know, because I've been there. You're trying to sneak in a workout with someone other than your "steady," and your former partner comes to do cardio. There is an uncomfortable silence and then the questions start:

"So, how long has this been going on?"…and "I suppose you've been doing lats behind my back, too?"

Then you have to defend yourself: "This is the only time, and it was an accident; it just happened. It meant nothing to me. We met at the juice bar and one set led to another. I was going to tell you…"

Before you know it, you've lost a good workout partner for one who has their own set of problems. The wheatgrass isn't always greener! To make matters worse, your old partner has moved on and now you have to see him or her training with someone else, and you can't find a tactful way to break up with the replacement. What do you say?

"I'm sorry, we're just not working out" or
"I don't feel like I'm growing with you" or
"I think I need to spot other people."

Having someone encourage, inspire, teach, or
guilt you into keeping up the fight can be an
important and fun way to make getting in shape a
reality. This is especially crucial with healthy
eating. Find someone to do it with you. If you are
married, try to get your other half on board, too,
because if someone eating beside you is having a
big bowl of something you love, you're going to
break down and order it, too.

Also avoid those people who make fun of how
you eat, until you're able to fend off peer pressure.
Idiot friends who call you "Mr. Salad" or "Ms.
On-the-side" can be the death of a slim-down
plan.

If you need to, be the first one to order a meal and
guilt everyone else into doing the right thing.
Your move, fatties!

It's never too late

If you are not currently exercising and eating right, there is no better time to start than NOW! A recent IRSA study showed that the biggest increase in gym memberships is in the 55-and-older group. It looks as though there's going to be a lot more gray in the gym than just on the sweatpants, which I find very encouraging. After living in a retirement town in Florida, I have been motivated for years by super-fit octogenarians. There are so many senior citizens pumping iron that we've practically changed the name of our club to "Old's Gym." It's the only gym in the country with a walker mill. Our members didn't *do* pull-ups, they wear them. It's…an assisted lifting facility. (Yes, I'm finished now!)

Taking care of your body can be like taking care of your car; put the right fuel into it, in the right amounts and keep it moving. A car that sits idle actually deteriorates faster than one that is driven regularly. By putting in the work at any age, you will add not just years to your life, but life to your years!

Chapter 8

Key Words

Throughout the book, I've made jokes about certain words and foods that by their very nature are obviously bad for us or contribute to our being overweight. To make certain those words won't be forgotten, I've taken the liberty of putting them, and a few more, into this handy study guide:

Angel Food vs. Devil's Food Cake The classic battle between good and evil. Head towards the Angel food cake, or your eating plan is going to hell. Easy enough?

Avoid anything that denotes a larger or extreme size This includes but is not limited to Whopper, Biggie, Ultimate, Mega, Gigundo, Mighty, Triple XL, Supersize, Family Size (unless you're with your family), or any other word that makes eating it seem like a personal challenge.

(Also, if you are promised a t-shirt or your name on a plaque for finishing the meal, just say no!)

Fried Soaked in a batter and dunked in boiling oil is delicious, but bad for your diet! Think about it; have you ever heard the word "fried" used in a good way? For example: "Hard week at work, I'm totally fried" and "I think the kid who delivered our pizza was fried" do not conjure up positive images.

Fried Addendum It gets worse if you add the words "Southern" or "country" to the word "fried." Both words imply that the food was fried first, and then topped with gravy!

Sides At most restaurants, this includes mashed potatoes, mac n' cheese, fries, and other items that should be avoided, because they will end up "on *your* sides." Whenever possible, go for the steamed vegetables (no butter), fruit, or rice (but not the "fried" rice).

Mayo They don't call it the Mayo Clinic for nothing. This is one time it's okay *not* to use a condiment.

Dressing The kinds we put on salads are usually nothing more than spoonfuls of fat. And In the case of holiday meals, "dressing" or stuffing is mostly fat *and* tons of carbohydrates. A good way to remember to be careful here is to visualize what you'll look and feel like when dressing and undressing, if you eat too much of either kind of "dressing."

Dressing addendum: Ranch What lives on a ranch? Pigs and cows. Think about it.

Caesar Salad A clump of wet leaves coated in oil and cheese, named after an obese Roman dictator.

Wedge Salad A triangle of iceberg lettuce, fatty dressing, and bacon bits, named after the act of picking our underpants out of our butts.

Chef Salad Show me a thin chef.

Iceberg The nutritionally empty lettuce used by most restaurants. What we put on it to make it taste good is our diet downfall. The *iceberg* is what sinks your chances of losing weight.

Lite, Lo-fat, or Lo-cal If the manufacturers couldn't take the time to spell the words completely, they probably didn't take the time to make the foods they describe either healthy or good tasting. Pass on these.

Reduced Fat Reduced from what? Yes, the reduced fat version of your favorite Ranch dressing might have half the calories of its full-fat counterpart, but probably still contains too much per serving, because 80-100% of its calories come from fat. So skip it or make it yourself; and, when eating it, order it *on the side*.

Stuffed Most of the time, this means either stuffed with cheese and fat or stuffed to be way bigger than it should be for one serving. Think about how you feel when you say, "I'm stuffed." Do you *really* want to be "stuffed"?

Loaded See "stuffed." You might want to be "loaded" once in a while, but it's never a good thing for your food to be. In the case of a potato, it means piled with sour cream, butter, cheese, and bacon bits. And, as opposed to popular thought, potatoes by themselves are not bad for you...until they're loaded.

Casseroles I looked this up and learned it is French for "food that goes straight to your butt." C'mon, it's got the word *ass* right in it! Almost every casserole recipe I've ever seen contains cream, butter, and cheese.

Trans-fats This is the RuPaul of diet and health mistakes. You think you're having a normal fat and, boom, it's a trans-fat. Without getting into science, trans-fats are chemically altered fats that don't occur naturally. If hearing that they are fats doesn't keep you away, then finding out that they are genetically modified fats definitely should.

Good Words

Skinny Thank you, coffee people! Order your coffee this way to cut the calories way down.

Baked "Fried" didn't work in a sentence, but "baked" fits nicely into most phrases. When ordering most foods, you also choose, broiled, grilled, steamed, or roasted. And remember, blackened does not mean burned.

Chapter 9

Whole Wheat or Not, It's a Wrap

Compliments for a comedian after a show come in varying degrees, starting with "I laughed so hard my cheeks hurt," moving up to "I laughed so hard I cried," and going all the way up to "I laughed so hard I think I peed a little." The same goes for fitness comedians, especially considering that the first two responses burned calories and the third one resulted in actual weight loss.

My goals for writing this book, aside from making you laugh, was for the information in it to help you unlearn some of the BS you may have heard over the years and to show you some easy ways to actually lose weight. "Easy" should be the most important truth you take away from all of this, because eating healthy and losing weight is really *not* that hard.

You can make moves as small as cutting back on sodas or reducing your cheese intake, and see big drop on the scale over time. Add a dash of exercise, and you may find that the weight falling off. Realistically, that is a great goal! A pound here or a pound there over a year or two can become 20, 30, or even 50 pounds that come off and stays off.

Start thinking about the words in everything you eat, like mayo=Mayo Clinic, and dressings should be on the side or they will end up on *your* side. Make good food decisions a part of your routine, and save cheat meals and treats for special occasions.

And all of those choices will keep you headed in the right direction, so you won't need to try some fad diet that makes your weight yo-yo. You remember playing with a yo-yo, don't you? It seemed really cool when that kid with no friends was able to make one do all those tricks, but when you tried to do that, it worked for a minute and then the string ended up in knots.

You are *not* a yo-yo. Common sense is more common than we give it credit for being. Trust your brain and gut, not your eyes and nose. The latter pair will lead you to the smell of donuts and pizza every time, even when the former pair tries to remind you about the weight gain, guilt, and indigestion you will suffer.

It's easy. You *can* do this. If laughing your abs off becomes difficult, I recommend a trip to your local comedy club once every two weeks. Hold your stomach tight, breathe deeply, and release, because if you try to hold laughs in, you'll fart.

Acknowledgements

I want to thank the following people:

My wife, Michelle, who inspired me to write, eat right, share with others, and (most important) chill out in the gym a little before I break something else; KB, my training partner and overall inspiration; and Cheryl, the surprising wealth of diet knowledge; and Carmen, my mentor, and the one who pushed me to blend my comedy and love of working out. Jan Tana for the elevator ride that launched a career; Debbie Baigrie for validating and encouraging some of my first fitness/comedy writing in *Natural Muscle Magazine*; Rob Wilkins, an inspiration in fitness and an all-around great American; Gene Schlossberg; Brian and Jen, who are both champions and great friends; Tim Gardner; Sandra Bishop at MacGregor Literary for believing in me every step of the way; Bobby

and Patricia Rossi, and all my friends at Ruth
Eckerd Hall;

Bill Parisi; Martin "Rambo" Rooney; Mark
Caruso from Sarasota GNC for supporting my
addictions; Bruce Day; Bob Wolff; Tad T. and
Gina for fostering serious ab-envy; Nick and Erik;
Jimmy P.; Bobby Jewell; Paul and Judy Deasy,
The Martin Brothers, Les and Pam McCurdy;
Sandi McKenna; Rene Harte; Jonathan Crespo;
Derek Scharlin; Philly; Ken Michelini; and Coach
SteveO/Steven Ledbetter for help beyond what I
could have asked for; my editor, Derry, who
corrected my total inability to use the English
language with more grace and red ink than a U.S.
budget proposal; Tres Cunningham, cover artist
extraordinaire; and Laree Draper, who went from
being the wife of one of my idols to being one of
my idols over the course of a few hundred
invaluable emails.

There are more than a few others who inspired me
along the way without knowing it; Ron Walker for
dragging me to the gym; Bill Phillips from EAS;

Clark Bartram, Chris Poirer, Gray Cook, Dan John, Tony Little, Victor Konavolov, Deke, Tony, Pete, and the NPC gang. Yes, I know the potato goes in the front; my drill instructors and years in the USMC for providing the spine; and countless others who either cheered for me or, at the very least, didn't tell me I couldn't!

And, of course, my parents and family, especially my sister Tracie. Thank you for supporting me through every dream, struggle, and idea, without ever saying no or telling me I was crazy!

www.ingramcontent.com/pod-product-compliance
Lightning Source LLC
Chambersburg PA
CBHW050118280326
41933CB00010B/1156